Mediterranean Recipes for Busy People

Super-Quick and Healthy Recipes to Save Your Time and Boost Your Meals

I0145896

America Best Recipes

Table of contents

Cucumber Rolls

Preparation Time: 5 minutes

Cooking Time: 0 minutes

Servings: 6

Ingredients:

- 1 big cucumber, sliced lengthwise
- 1 tbsp. parsley, chopped
- 8 oz. canned tuna, drained and mashed
- Salt and black pepper to the taste
- 1 tsp. lime juice

Directions:

- Arrange cucumber slices on a working surface, divide the rest of the ingredients, and roll.
- Arrange all the rolls on a platter and serve as an appetizer.

Nutrition:

Calories 200;

Fat 6 g;

Carbs 7.6 g;

Protein 3.5 g

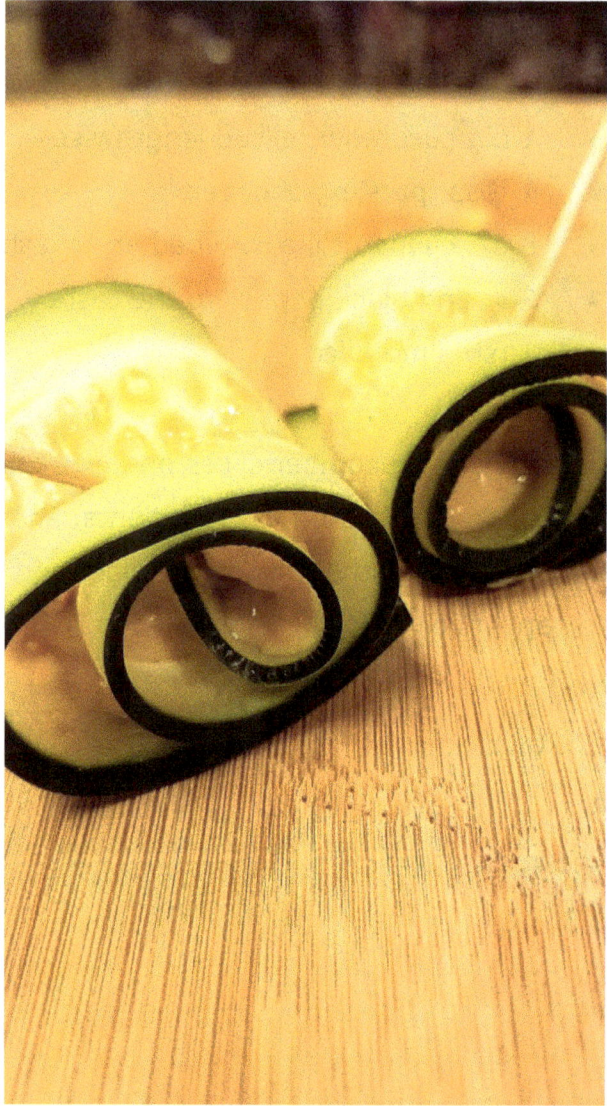

Olives and Cheese Stuffed Tomatoes

Preparation Time: 10 minutes

Cooking Time: 0 minutes

Servings: 24

Ingredients :

- 24 cherry tomatoes, top cut off and insides scooped out
- 2 tbsp. olive oil
- ¼ tsp. red pepper flakes
- ½ cup feta cheese, crumbled
- 2 tbsp. black olive paste
- ¼ cup mint, torn

Directions:

1. In a bowl, mix the olives paste with the rest of the ingredients except the cherry tomatoes and whisk well. Stuff the cherry tomatoes with this mix, arrange them all on a platter and serve as an appetizer.

Nutrition:

Calories 136;

Fat 8.6 g;

Carbs 5.6 g;

Protein 5.1 g

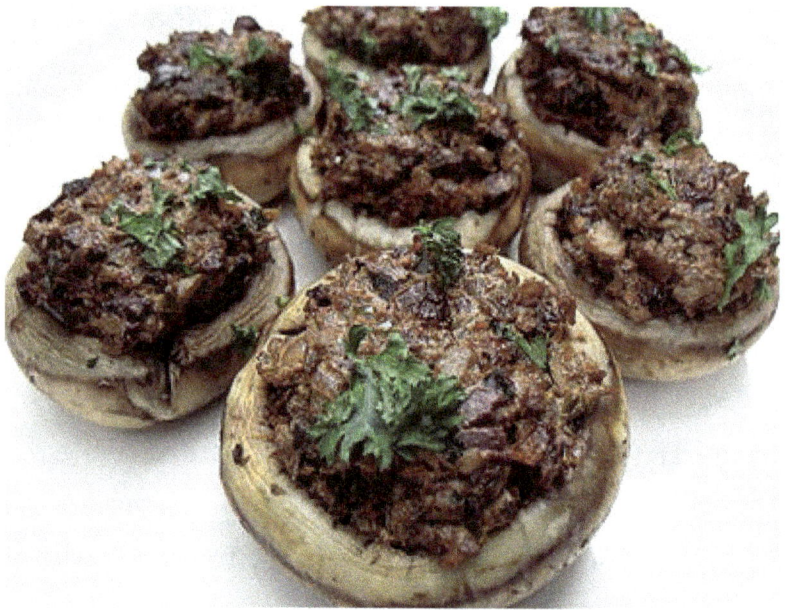

Tomato Salsa

Preparation Time: 5 minutes

Cooking Time: 0 minutes

Servings: 6

Ingredients:

- 1 garlic clove, minced
- 4 tbsp. olive oil
- 5 tomatoes, cubed
- 1 tbsp. balsamic vinegar
- ¼ cup basil, chopped
- 1 tbsp. parsley, chopped
- 1 tbsp. chives, chopped
- Salt and black pepper to the taste
- Pita chips for serving

Directions:

1. In a bowl, mix the tomatoes with the garlic and the rest of the ingredients except the pita chips, stir, divide into small cups and serve with the pita chips on the side.

Nutrition:

Calories 160;

Fat 13.7 g;

Carbs 10.1 g;

Protein 2.2

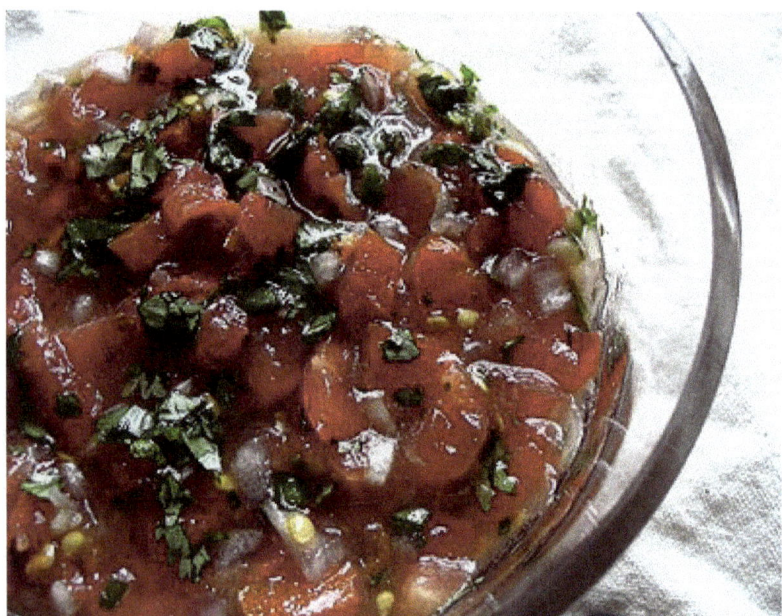

Chili Mango and Watermelon Salsa

Preparation Time: 5 minutes

Cooking Time: 0 minutes

Servings: 12

Ingredients :

- 1 red tomato, chopped
- Salt and black pepper to the taste
- 1 cup watermelon, seedless, peeled and cubed
- 1 red onion, chopped
- 2 mangos, peeled and chopped
- 2 chili peppers, chopped
- ¼ cup cilantro, chopped
- 3 tbsp. lime juice
- Pita chips for serving

Directions:

1. In a bowl, mix the tomato with the watermelon, the onion and the rest of the ingredients except the pita chips and toss well. Divide the mix into small cups and serve with pita chips on the side.

Nutrition:

Calories 62;

Fat 2g;

Fiber 1.3 g;

Carbs 3.9 g;

Protein 2.3 g

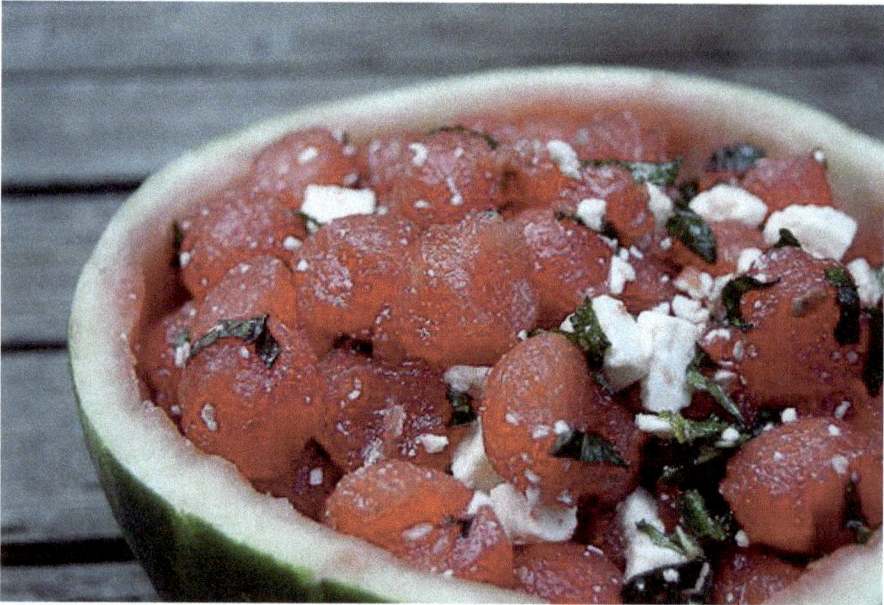

Creamy Spinach and Shallots Dip

Preparation Time: 10 minutes

Cooking Time: 0 minutes

Servings: 4

Ingredients:

1. 1 lb. spinach, roughly chopped
2. 2 shallots, chopped
3. 2 tbsp. mint, chopped
4. ¾ cup cream cheese, soft
5. Salt and black pepper to the taste

Directions:

1. In a blender, combine the spinach with the shallots and the rest of the ingredients, and pulse well. Divide into small bowls and serve as a party dip.

Nutrition:

Calories 204;

Fat 11.5 g;

Carbs 4.2 g;

Protein 5.9 g

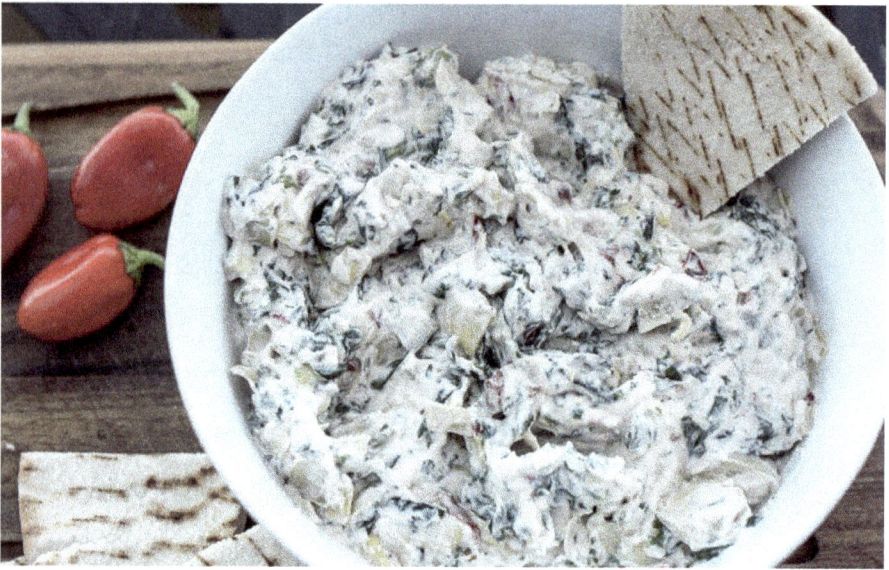

Feta Artichoke Dip

Preparation Time: 10 minutes

Cooking Time: 30 minutes

Servings: 8

Ingredients:

- 8 oz. artichoke hearts, drained and quartered
- ¾ cup basil, chopped
- ¾ cup green olives, pitted and chopped
- 1 cup parmesan cheese, grated
- 5 oz. feta cheese, crumbled

Directions:

1. In your food processor, mix the artichokes with the basil and the rest of the ingredients, pulse well, and transfer to a baking dish.
2. Introduce in the oven, bake at 375° F for 30 minutes and serve as a party dip.

Nutrition:

Calories 186;

Fat 12.4 g;

Fiber 0.9 g;

Carbs 2.6 g;

Protein 1.5 g

Avocado Dip

Preparation Time: 5 minutes

Cooking Time: 0 minutes

Servings: 8

Ingredients:

- ½ cup heavy cream
- 1 green chili pepper, chopped
- Salt and pepper to the taste
- 4 avocados, pitted, peeled and chopped
- 1 cup cilantro, chopped
- ¼ cup lime juice

Directions:

- In a blender, combine the cream with the avocados and the rest of the ingredients and pulse well. Divide the mix into bowls and serve cold as a party dip.

Nutrition:

Calories 200;

Fat 14.5 g;

Fiber 3.8 g;

Carbs 8.1 g;

Protein 7.6 g

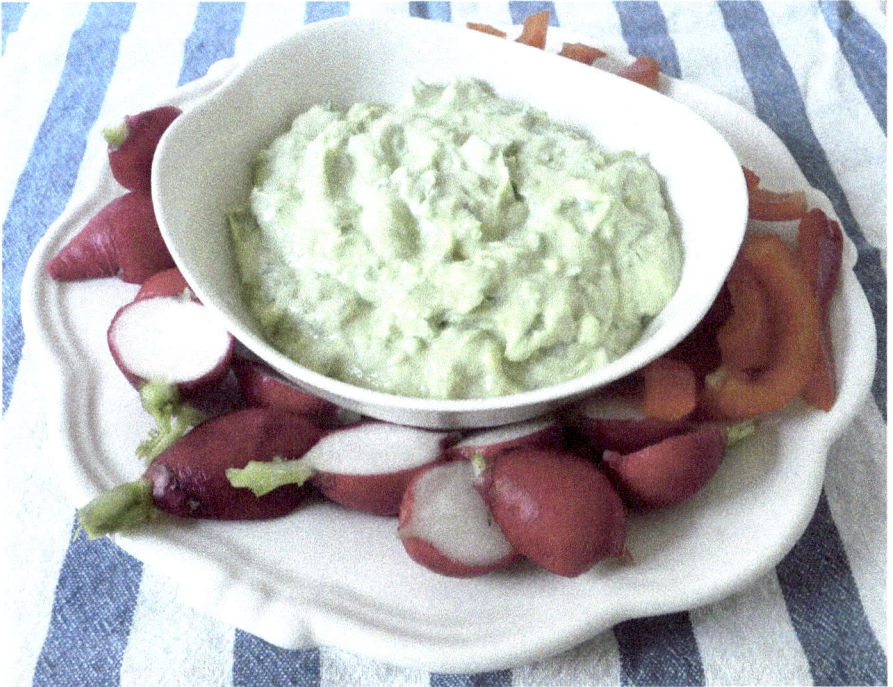

Goat Cheese and Chives Spread

Preparation Time: 10 minutes

Cooking Time: 0 minute

Servings: 4

Ingredients :

1. 2 oz. goat cheese, crumbled
2. ¾ cup sour cream
3. 2 tbsp. chives, chopped
4. 1 tbsp. lemon juice
5. Salt and black pepper to the taste
6. 2 tbsp. extra virgin olive oil

Directions:

1. In a bowl, mix the goat cheese with the cream and the rest of the ingredients and whisk really well. Keep in the fridge for 10 minutes and serve as a party spread.

Nutrition:

Calories 220;

Fat 11.5 g;

Carbs 8.9 g;

Protein 5.6 g

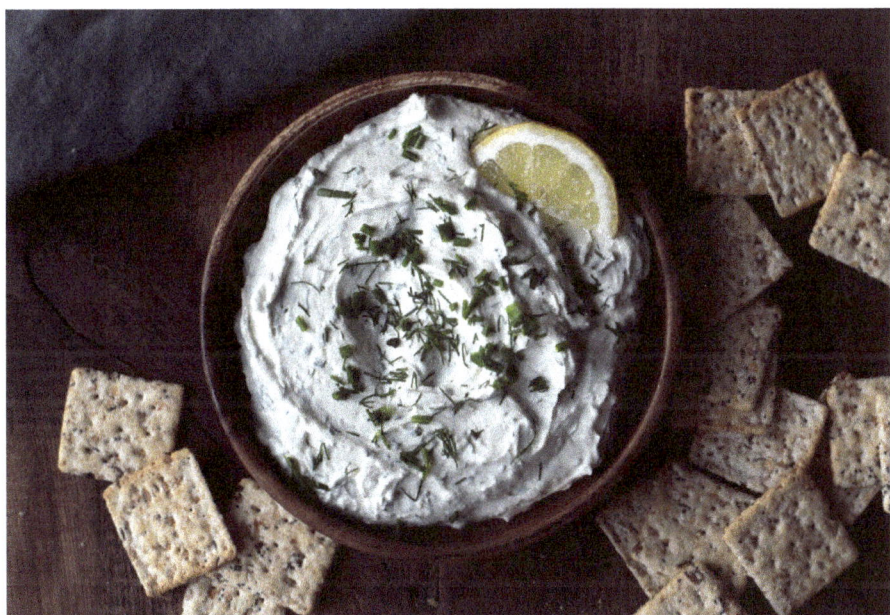

Stuffed Chicken

Preparation Time: 10 minutes

Cooking Time: 30 minutes

Serves: 4

Ingredients:

- 4 chicken breasts, skinless, boneless and butterflied
- 1 oz. spring onions, chopped
- ½ lb. white mushrooms, sliced
- 1 tsp. hot paprika
- A pinch of salt and black pepper
- 1 cup tomato sauce

Directions:

2. Flatten chicken breasts with a meat mallet and place them on a plate.
3. In a bowl, mix the spring onions with the mushrooms, paprika, salt and pepper and stir well.
4. Divide this on each chicken breast half, roll them and secure with a toothpick.
5. Add the tomato sauce in the instant pot, put the chicken rolls inside as well. put the lid on and cook on High for 30 minutes.

6. Release the pressure naturally for 10 minutes, arrange the stuffed chicken breasts on a platter and serve.

Nutrition:

Calories 221,

Fat 12g,

Carbs 6g,

Protein 11g

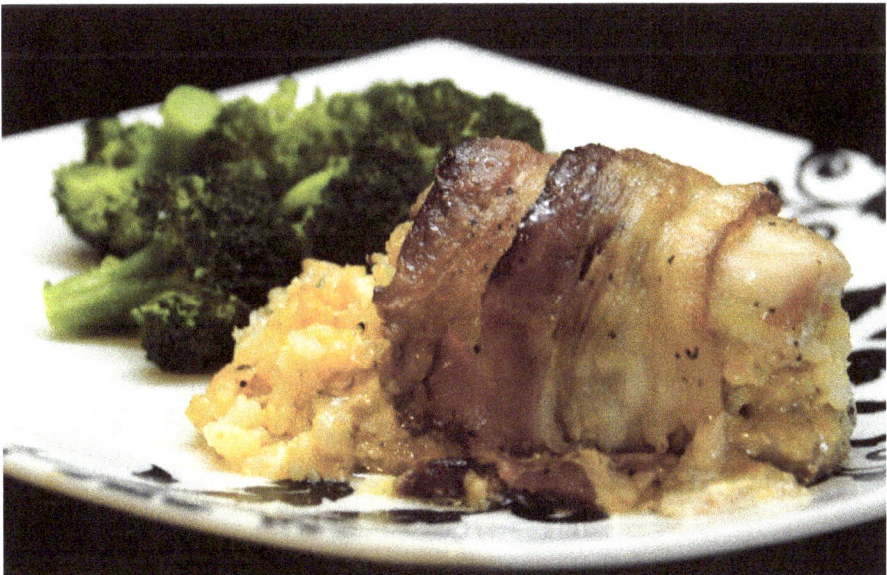

Cinnamon Baby Black Ribs Platter

Preparation Time: 10 minutes

Cooking Time: 40 minutes

Serves: 2

Ingredients:

1. 1 rack baby back ribs
2. 2 tsp. smoked paprika
3. 2 tsp. chili powder
4. A pinch of salt and black pepper
5. 1 tsp. garlic powder
6. 1 tsp. onion powder
7. 1 tsp. cinnamon powder
8. ½ tsp. cumin seeds
9. A pinch of cayenne pepper
10. 1 cup tomato sauce
11. 3 garlic cloves, minced

Directions:

- In your instant pot, combine the baby back ribs with the rest of the ingredients, put the lid on and cook on High for 30 minutes.
- Release the pressure naturally for 10 minutes, arrange the ribs on a platter and serve as an appetizer.

Nutrition:

Calories 222,

Fat 12g,

Fiber 4g,

Carbs 6g,

Protein 14g

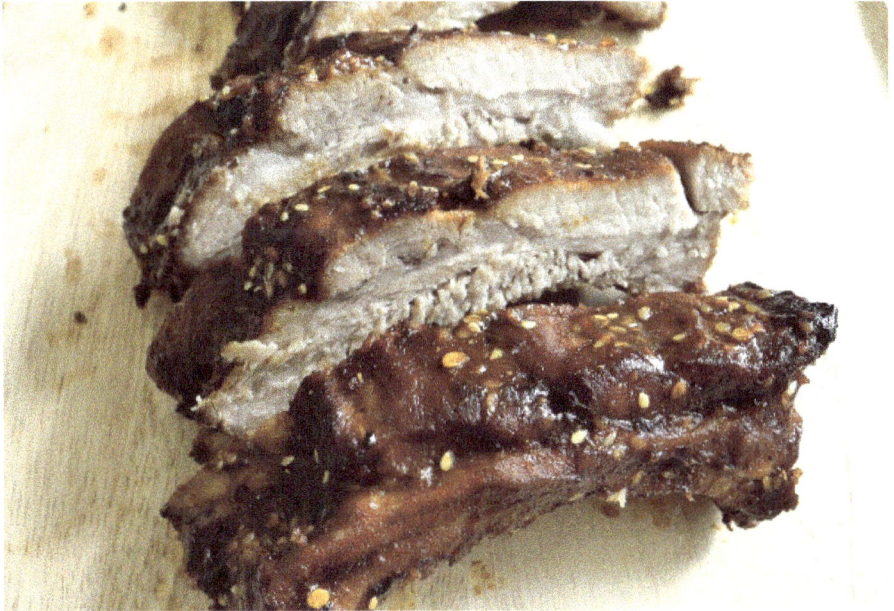

Buttery Carrot Sticks

Preparation Time: 10 minutes

Cooking Time: 15 minutes

Serves: 4

Ingredients:

1. 1 lb. carrot, cut into sticks
2. 4 garlic cloves, minced
3. ¼ cup chicken stock
4. 1 tsp. rosemary, chopped
5. A pinch of salt and black pepper
6. 2 tbsp. olive oil
7. 2 tbsp. ghee, melted

Directions:

- Set the instant pot on Sauté mode, add the oil and the ghee, heat them up, add the garlic and brown for 1 minute.
- Add the rest of the ingredients, put the lid on and cook on High for 14 minutes.
- Release the pressure naturally for 10 minutes, arrange the carrot sticks on a platter and serve.

Nutrition:

Calories 142,

Fat 4g,

Carbs 5g,

Protein 7g

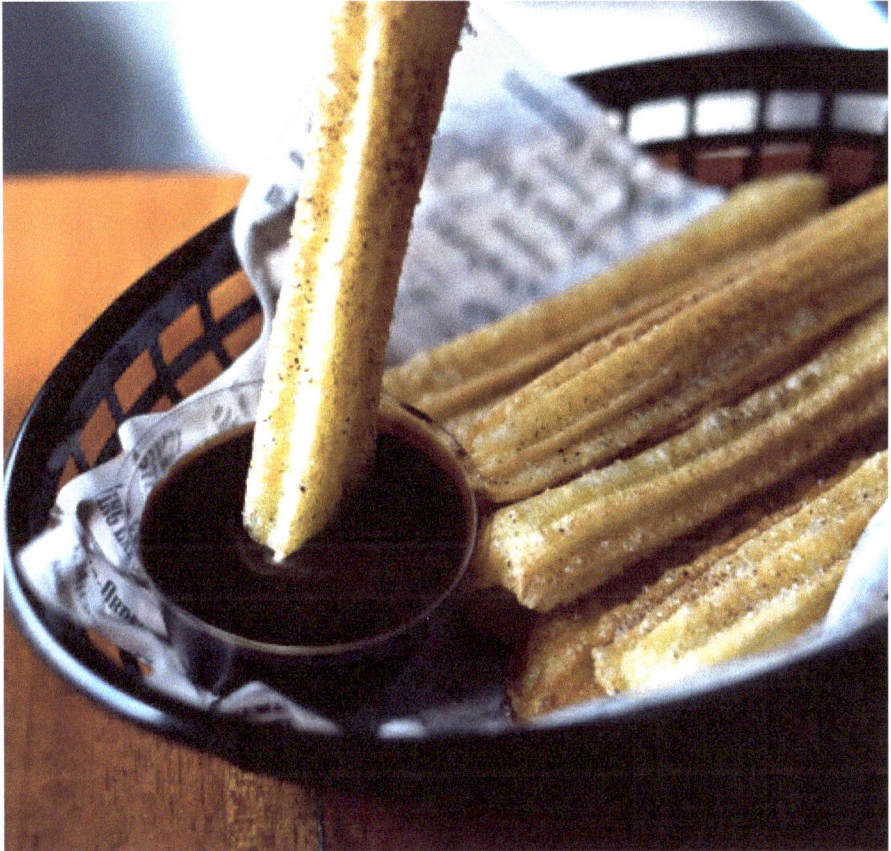

Cajun Walnuts And Olives Bowls

Preparation Time: 10 minutes

Cooking Time: 10 minutes

Serves: 2

Ingredients:

1. ½ lb. walnuts, chopped
2. A pinch of salt and black pepper
3. 1 and ½ cups black olives, pitted
4. ½ tbsp. Cajun seasoning
5. 2 garlic cloves, minced
6. 1 red chili pepper, chopped
7. ¼ cup veggie stock
8. 2 tbsp. tomato puree

Directions:

- In your instant pot, combine the walnuts with the olives and the rest of the ingredients, put the lid on and cook on High 10 minutes.
- Release the pressure fast for 5 minutes, divide the mix into small bowls and serve as an appetizer.

Nutrition:

Calories 105,

Fat 1g,

Fiber 1g,

Carbs 4g,

Protein 7g

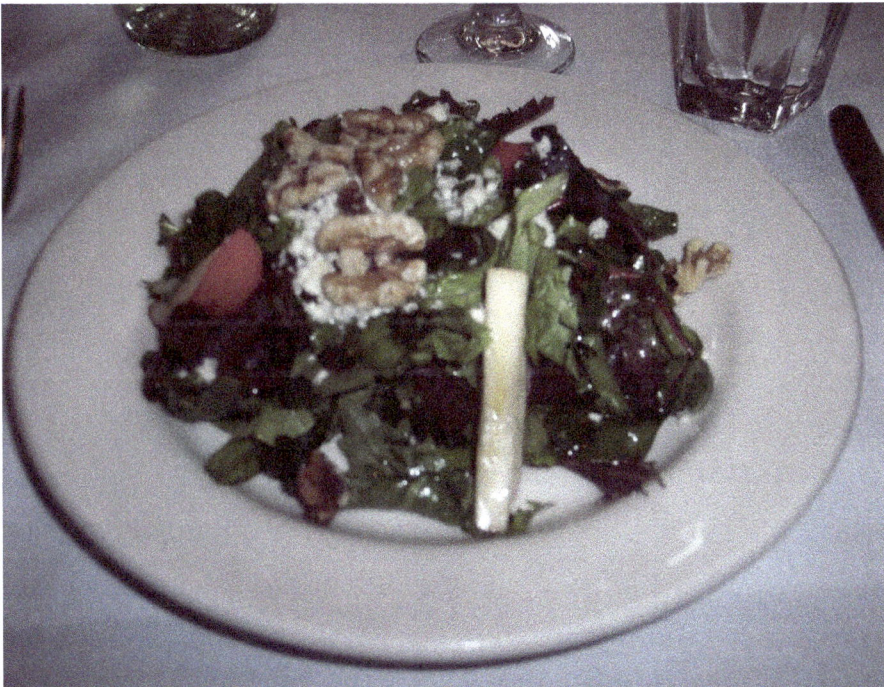

Mango Salsa

Preparation Time: 10 minutes

Cooking Time: 10 minutes

Serves: 2

Ingredients:

1. 2 mangoes, peeled and cubed
2. ½ tbsp. sweet paprika
3. 2 garlic cloves, minced
4. 2 tbsp. cilantro, chopped
5. 1 tbsp. spring onions, chopped
6. 1 cup cherry tomatoes, cubed
7. 1 cup avocado, peeled, pitted and cubed
8. A pinch of salt and black pepper
9. 1 tbsp. olive oil
10. ¼ cup tomato puree
11. ½ cup kalamata olives, pitted and sliced

Directions:

- In your instant pot, combine the mangoes with the paprika and the rest of the ingredients except the cilantro, put the lid on and cook on High for 5 minutes.
- Release the pressure fast for 5 minutes, divide the mix into small bowls, sprinkle the cilantro on top and serve.

Nutrition:

Calories 123,

Fat 4g,

Carbs 3g,

Protein 5g

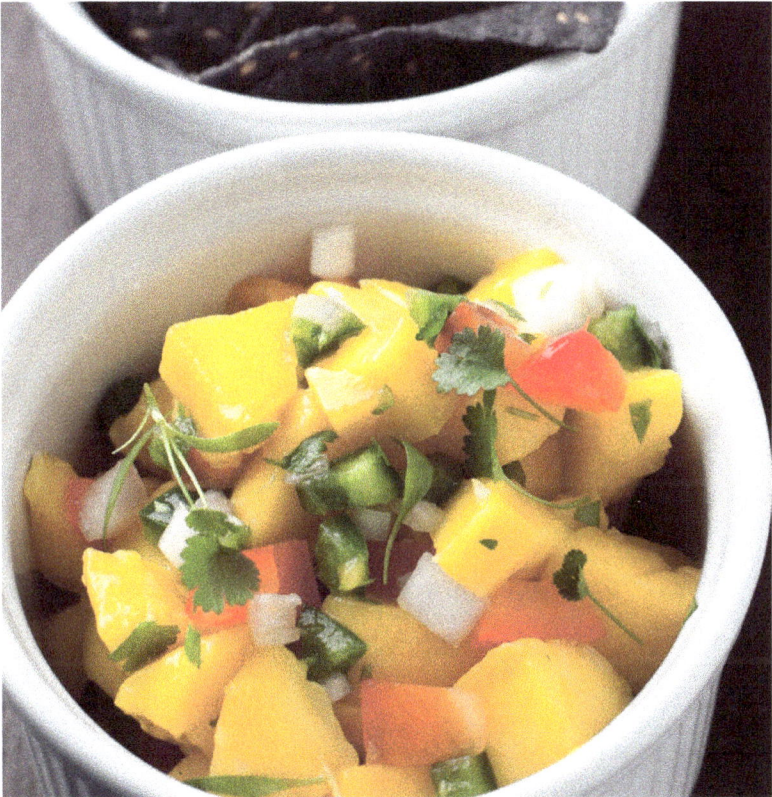

Hot Asparagus Sticks

Preparation Time: 10 minutes

Cooking Time: 10 minutes

Serves: 2

Ingredients:

1. 1 and ½ lb. asparagus, trimmed
2. 2 tbsp. olive oil
3. 2 tbsp. cayenne pepper sauce
4. A pinch of salt and black pepper
5. 1 cup water

Directions:

- In a bowl, mix the asparagus with the other ingredients except the water and toss.
- Put the water in your instant pot, add the steamer basket, put the asparagus sticks inside, put the lid on and cook on High for 6 minutes.
- Release the pressure fast for 5 minutes, arrange the asparagus on a platter and serve.

Nutrition:

Calories 181,

Fat 6g,

Carbs 4g,

Protein 4g

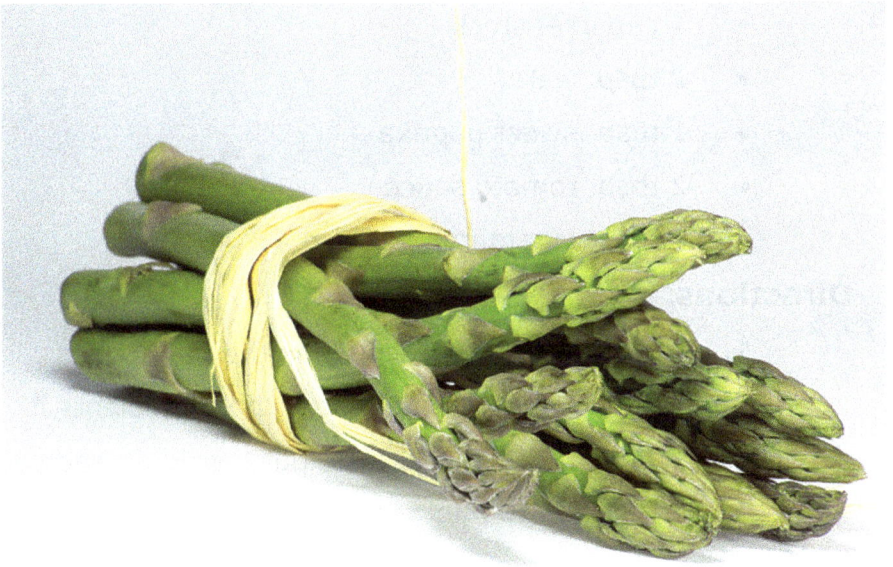

Pork Bites

Preparation Time: 10 minutes

Cooking Time: 30 minutes

Serves: 4

Ingredients:

- 1 lb. pork roast, cubed and browned
- 1 tbsp. Italian seasoning
- 1 cup beef stock
- 2 tbsp. water
- 1 tbsp. sweet paprika
- 2 tbsp. tomato sauce
- 1 tbsp. rosemary, chopped

Directions:

1. In your instant pot, combine the pork cubes with the seasoning and the rest of the ingredients except the rosemary, toss, put the lid on and cook on High for 30 minutes.
2. Release the pressure naturally for 10 minutes, arrange the pork cubes on a platter, sprinkle the rosemary on top and serve.

Nutrition:

Calories 242,

Fat 12g,

Carbs 6g,

Protein 14g

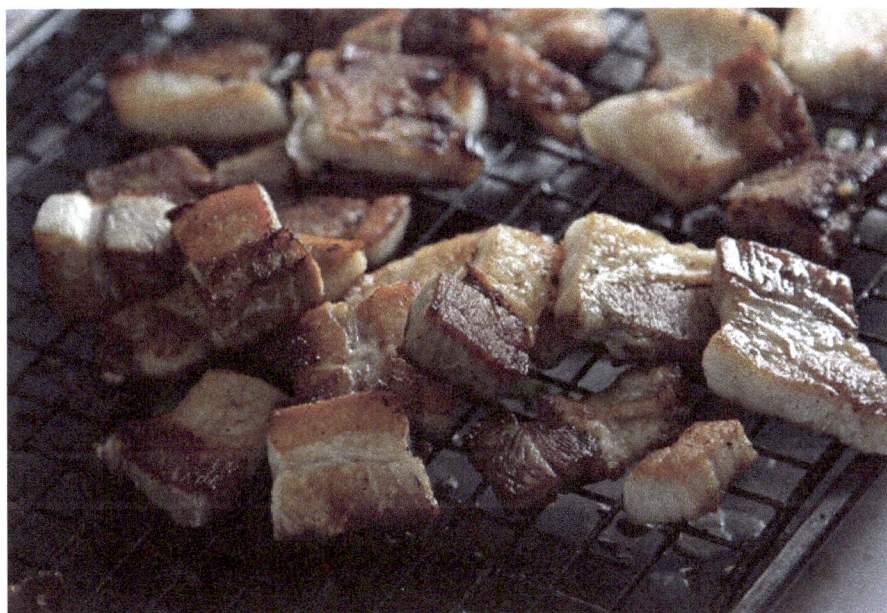

Meatballs Platter

Preparation Time: 10 minutes

Cooking Time: 15 minutes

Servings: 4

Ingredients:

- 1 lb. beef meat, ground
- ¼ cup panko breadcrumbs
- A pinch of salt and black pepper
- 3 tbsp. red onion, grated
- ¼ cup parsley, chopped
- 2 garlic cloves, minced
- 2 tbsp. lemon juice
- Zest of 1 lemon, grated
- 1 egg
- ½ tsp. cumin, ground
- ½ tsp. coriander, ground
- ¼ tsp. cinnamon powder
- 2 oz. feta cheese, crumbled

Directions:

1.   In a bowl, mix the beef with the breadcrumbs, salt, pepper and the rest of the ingredients except the cooking spray, stir well and shape medium balls out of this mix.

2. Arrange the meatballs on a baking sheet lined with parchment paper, grease them with cooking spray and bake at 450°F for 15 minutes.
3. Arrange the meatballs on a platter and serve as an appetizer.

Nutrition:

Calories 300;

Fat 15.4 g;

Carbs 22.4 g;

Protein 35 g

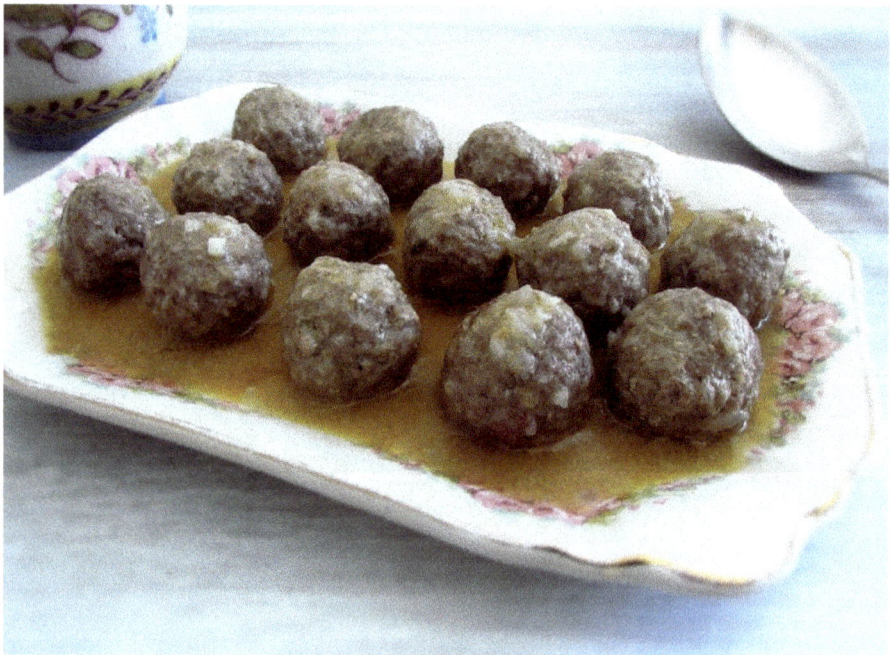

Yogurt Dip

Preparation Time: 10 minutes

Cooking Time: 0 minutes

Servings: 6

Ingredients:

- 2 cups Greek yogurt
- 2 tbsp. pistachios, toasted and chopped
- A pinch of salt and white pepper
- 2 tbsp. mint, chopped
- 1 tbsp. kalamata olives, pitted and chopped
- ¼ cup za'atar spice
- ¼ cup pomegranate seeds
- 1/3 cup olive oil

Directions:

1. In a bowl, combine the yogurt with the pistachios and the rest of the ingredients, whisk well, divide into small cups and serve with pita chips on the side.

Nutrition:

Calories 294;

Fat 18 g;

Carbs 21 g;

Protein 10 g

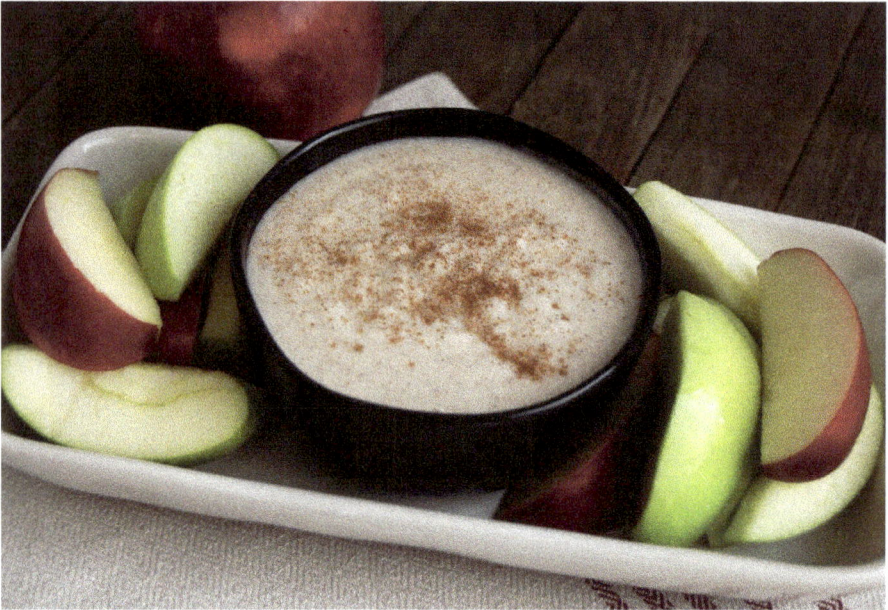

Tomato Bruschetta

Preparation Time: 10 minutes

Cooking Time: 10 minutes

Servings: 6

Ingredients:

- 1 baguette, sliced
- 1/3 cup basil, chopped
- 6 tomatoes, cubed
- 2 garlic cloves, minced
- A pinch of salt and black pepper
- 1 tsp. olive oil
- 1 tbsp. balsamic vinegar
- ½ tsp. garlic powder
- Cooking spray

Directions:

1. Arrange the baguette slices on a baking sheet lined with parchment paper, grease them with cooking spray and bake at 400° F for 10 minutes.
2. In a bowl, mix the tomatoes with the basil and the remaining ingredients, toss well and leave aside for 10 minutes.
3. Divide the tomato mix on each baguette slice, arrange them all on a platter and serve.

Nutrition:

Calories 162;

Fat 4 g;

Fiber 7 g;

Carbs 29 g;

Protein 4 g

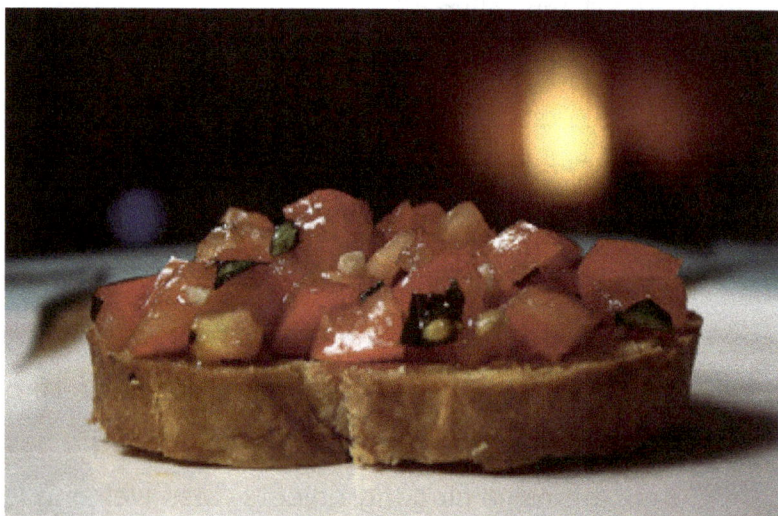

Artichoke Flatbread

Preparation Time: 10 minutes

Cooking Time: 15 minutes

Servings: 4

Ingredients:

- 5 tbsp. olive oil
- 2 garlic cloves, minced
- 2 tbsp. parsley, chopped
- 2 round whole wheat flatbreads
- 4 tbsp. parmesan, grated
- ½ cup mozzarella cheese, grated
- 14 oz. canned artichokes, drained and quartered
- 1 cup baby spinach, chopped
- ½ cup cherry tomatoes, halved
- ½ tsp. basil, dried
- Salt and black pepper to the taste

Directions:

1. In a bowl, mix the parsley with the garlic and 4 tbsp. oil, whisk well and spread this over the flatbreads.
2. Sprinkle the mozzarella and half of the parmesan.
3. In a bowl, mix the artichokes with the spinach, tomatoes, basil, salt, pepper and the rest of the oil, toss and divide over the flatbreads as well.
4. Sprinkle the rest of the parmesan on top, arrange the flatbreads on a baking sheet lined with

parchment paper and bake at 425° F for 15 minutes.

5.   Serve as an appetizer.

Nutrition:

Calories 223;

Fat 11.2 g;

Carbs 15.5 g;

Protein 7.4 g

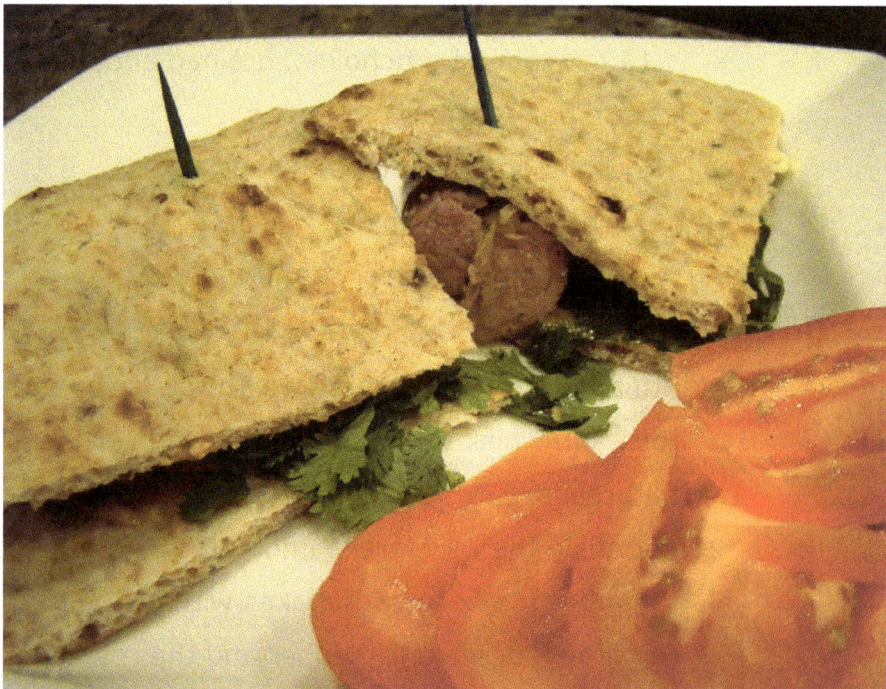

Red Pepper Tapenade

Preparation Time: 10 minutes

Cooking Time: 0 minutes

Servings: 4

Ingredients:

- 7 oz. roasted red peppers, chopped
- ½ cup parmesan, grated
- 1/3 cup parsley, chopped
- 14 oz. canned artichokes, drained and chopped
- 3 tbsp. olive oil
- ¼ cup capers, drained
- 1 and ½ tbsp. lemon juice
- 2 garlic cloves, minced

Directions:

1. In your blender, combine the red peppers with the parmesan and the rest of the ingredients and pulse well.
2. Divide into cups and serve as a snack.

Nutrition:

Calories 200;

Fat 5.6 g;

Carbs 12.4 g;

Protein 4.6 g

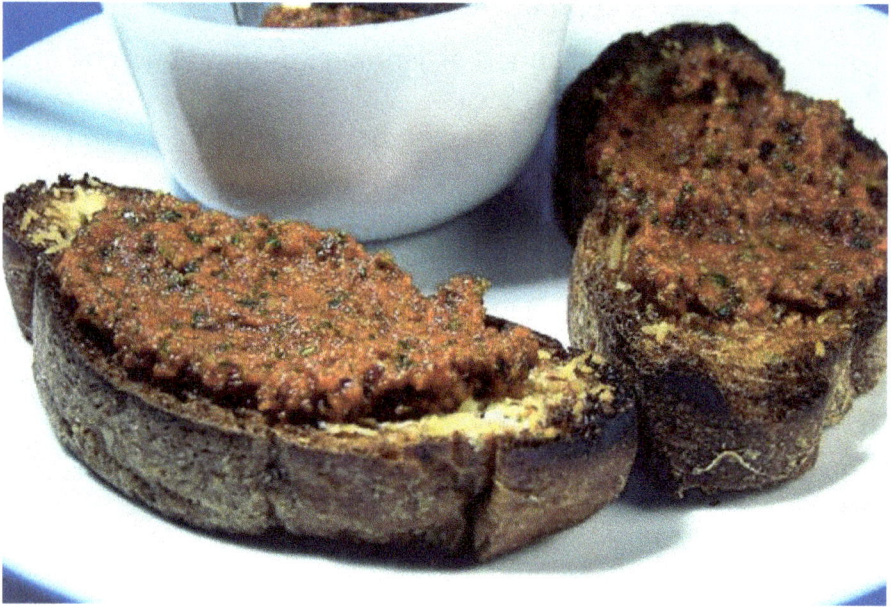

Coriander Falafel

Preparation Time: 10 minutes

Cooking Time: 10 minutes

Servings: 8

Ingredients:

- 1 cup canned garbanzo beans, drained and rinsed
- 1 bunch parsley leaves
- 1 yellow onion, chopped
- 5 garlic cloves, minced
- 1 tsp. coriander, ground
- A pinch of salt and black pepper
- ¼ tsp. cayenne pepper
- ¼ tsp. baking soda
- ¼ tsp. cumin powder
- 1 tsp. lemon juice
- 3 tbsp. tapioca flour
- Olive oil for frying

Directions:

1. In your food processor, combine the beans with the parsley, onion and the rest the ingredients except the oil and the flour and pulse well.
2. Transfer the mix to a bowl, add the flour, stir well, shape 16 balls out of this mix and flatten them a bit.

3. Heat up a pan with some oil over medium-high
   heat, add the falafels, cook them for 5 minutes on
   each side, transfer to paper towels, drain excess
   grease, arrange them on a platter and serve as an
   appetizer.

Nutrition:

Calories 112;

Fat 6.2 g;

Carbs 12.3 g;

Protein 3.1g

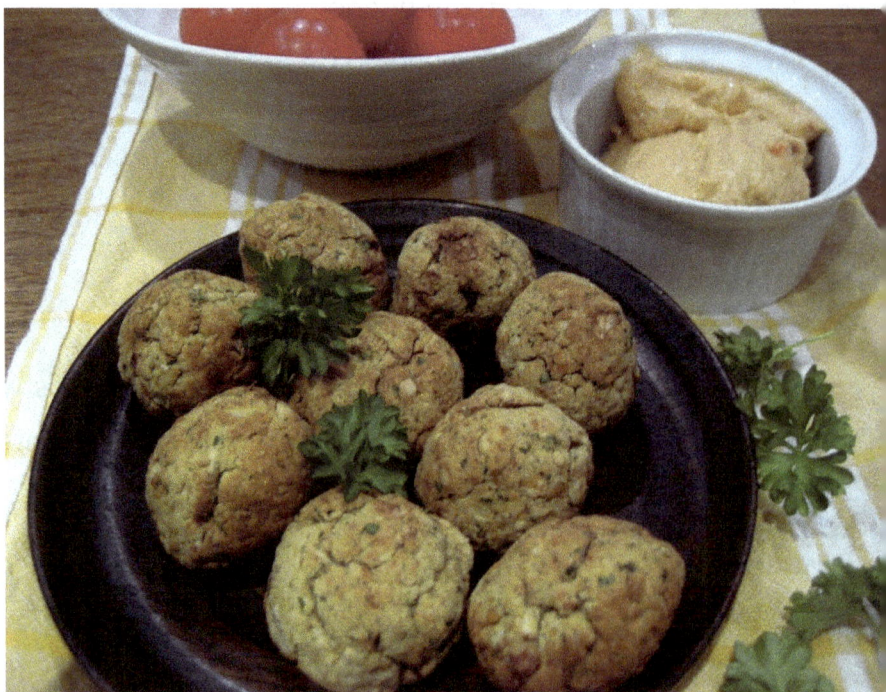

Red Pepper Hummus

Preparation Time: 10 minutes

Cooking Time: 0 minutes

Servings: 6

Ingredients:

- 6 oz. roasted red peppers, peeled and chopped
- 16 oz. canned chickpeas, drained and rinsed
- ¼ cup Greek yogurt
- 3 tbsp. tahini paste
- Juice of 1 lemon
- 3 garlic cloves, minced 1 tbsp. olive oil
- A pinch of salt and black pepper
- 1 tbsp. parsley, chopped

Directions:

1. In your food processor, combine the red peppers with the rest of the ingredients except the oil and the parsley and pulse well.
2. Add the oil, pulse again, divide into cups, sprinkle the parsley on top and serve as a party spread.

Nutrition:

Calories 255;

Fat 11.4 g;

Carbs 17.4 g;

Protein 6.5 g

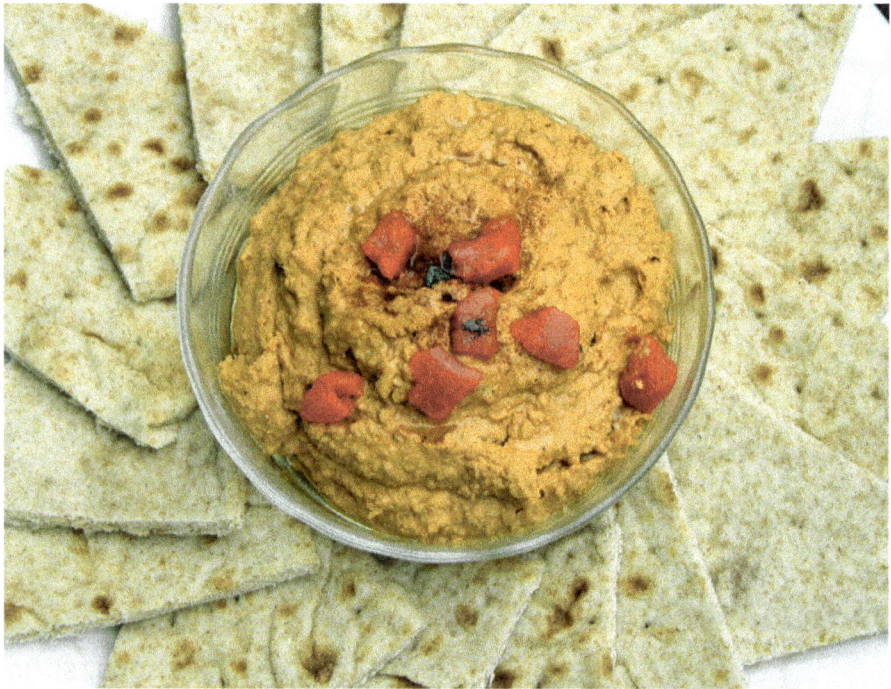

White Pizza with Prosciutto and Arugula

Preparation Time: 10 minutes

Cooking Time: 15 minutes

Servings: 6

Ingredients:

- 1 lb. prepared pizza dough
- ½ cup ricotta cheese
- 1 tbsp. garlic, minced
- 1 cup grated mozzarella cheese
- 3 oz. prosciutto, thinly sliced
- ½ cup fresh arugula
- ½ tsp. freshly ground black pepper

Directions:

1. Preheat the oven to 450°F. Roll out the pizza dough on a floured surface.
2. Put the pizza dough on a parchment-lined baking sheet or pizza sheet. Put the dough in the oven and bake for 8 minutes.
3. In a small bowl, mix together the ricotta, garlic, and mozzarella.
4. Remove the pizza dough from the oven and spread the cheese mixture over the top. Bake for another 5 to 6 minutes.

5. Top the pizza with prosciutto, arugula, and pepper; serve warm.

Nutrition:

Calories: 273;

Protein: 12.3g;

Carbs: 34g;

Fat: 11g

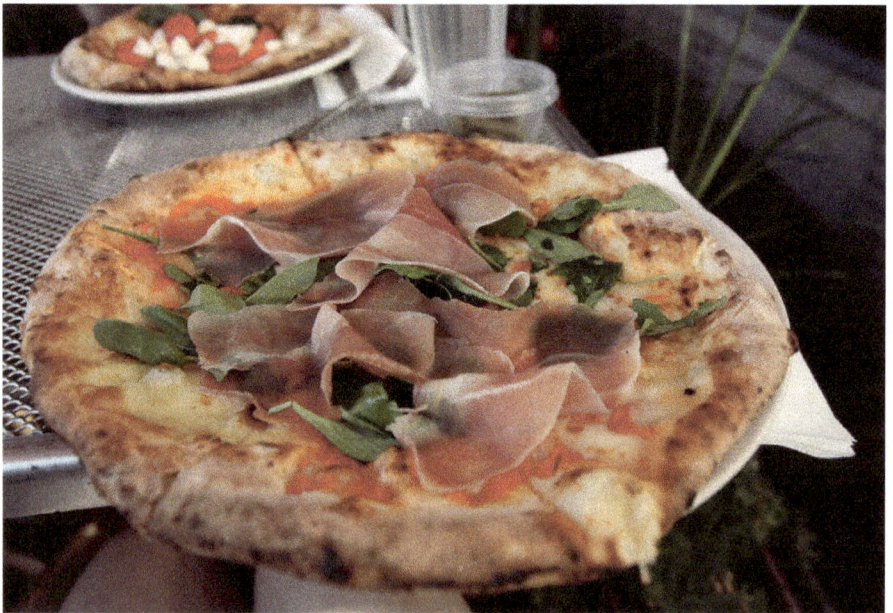

Za'atar Pizza

Preparation Time: 10 minutes

Cooking Time: 15 minutes

Servings: 5

Ingredients:

- 1 sheet puff pastry
- ¼ cup extra-virgin olive oil
- 1/3 cup za'atar seasoning

Directions:

1. Preheat the oven to 350°F.
2. Put the puff pastry on a parchment-lined baking sheet. Cut the pastry into desired slices.
3. Brush the pastry with olive oil. Sprinkle with the za'atar.
4. Put the pastry in the oven and bake for 10 to 12 minutes or until edges are lightly browned and puffed up. Serve warm or at room temperature.

Nutrition:

Calories: 153;

Protein: 10.3g;

Carbs: 21g;

Fat: 10g

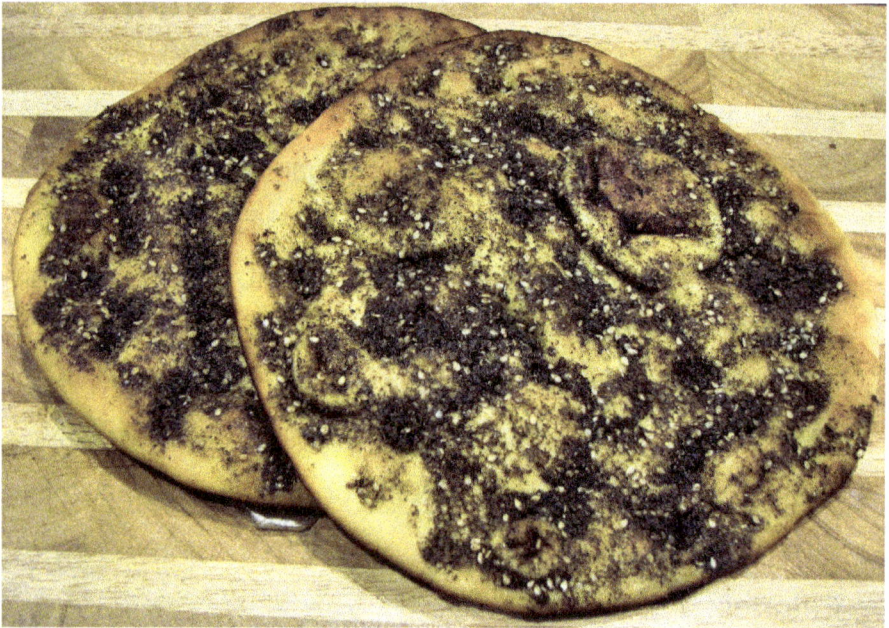

Broccoli Cheese Burst Pizza

Preparation Time: 20 minutes

Cooking Time: 5 minutes

Servings: 6

Ingredients:

- 1 cup mozzarella cheese, shredded
- 2/3 cup ricotta cheese
- 2 tsp. avocado oil
- 1 large whole-wheat pizza crust
- ¼ cup basil, chopped
- 1 ½ cups broccoli florets, chopped
- ½ tsp. garlic powder
- Cornmeal (for dusting)
- 1 ½ cups corn kernels
- Ground black pepper and salt, to taste

Directions:

1. Preheat your oven at 400°F. Take a baking sheet, line it with parchment paper. Grease it with some avocado oil. (You can also use cooking spray)
2. Spread some cornmeal over the baking sheet
3. In a mixing bowl, combine the corn, broccoli, ricotta, mozzarella, scallions, garlic powder, basil, black pepper and salt.

4. Place the pizza crust on the baking sheet. Add the topping mixture on top and bake until the top is light brown, for 12-15 minutes.
5. Slice and serve warm!

Nutrition: Calories – 417|Fat – 11g |Carbs – 53g |Fiber – 8|Protein – 19g

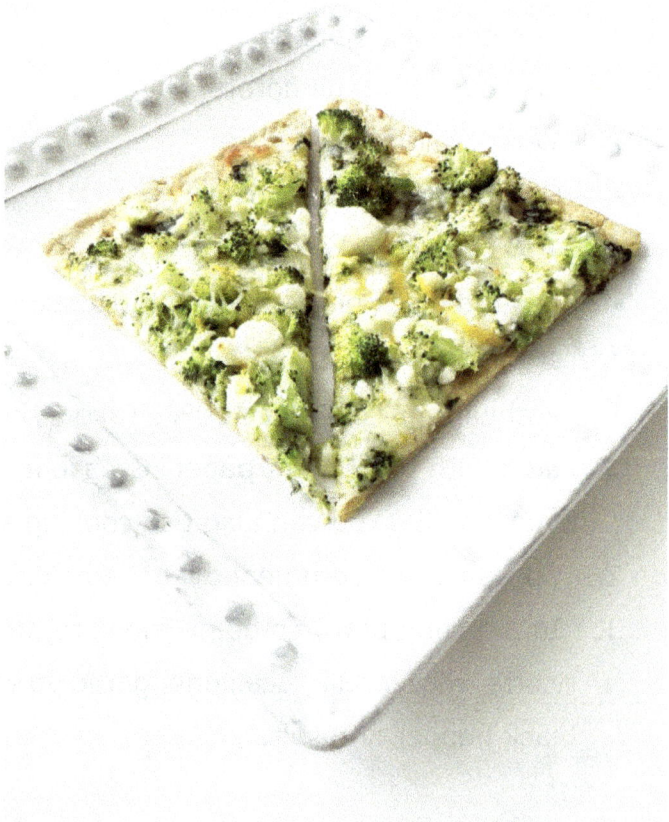

Mozzarella Bean Pizza

Preparation Time: 10 minutes

Cooking Time: 15 minutes

Servings: 6

Ingredients:

- 2 tbsp. cornmeal
- 1 cup mozzarella
- 1/3 cup barbecue sauce
- 1 roma tomato, diced
- 1 cup black beans
- 1 cup corn kernels
- 1 medium whole-wheat pizza crust

Directions:

1. Preheat your oven at 400°F. Take a baking sheet, line it with parchment paper. Grease it with some avocado oil. (You can also use cooking spray)
2. Spread some cornmeal over the baking sheet
3. In a bowl, mix together the tomatoes, corn and beans.
4. Place the pizza crust on the baking sheet. Spread the sauce on top; add the topping, and top with the cheese and bake until the cheese melts and the crust edges are golden-brown for 12-15 minutes.
5. Slice and serve warm.

Nutrition: Calories – 223 |Fat – 14g|Carbs – 41g|Fiber – 6g|Protein – 8g

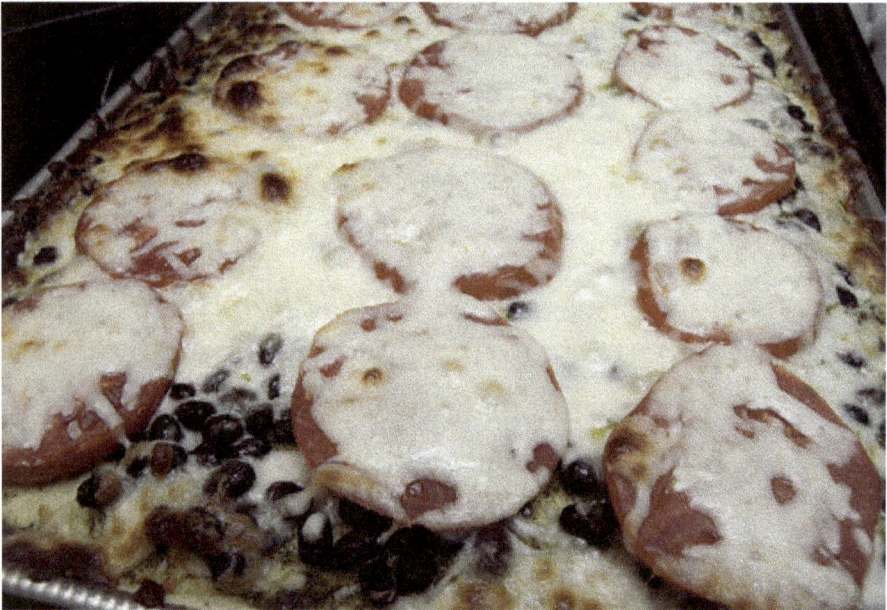

Olive Oil Pizza Dough

Preparation Time: 10 minutes

Cooking Time: 15 minutes

Servings: 5

Ingredients:

- Water 2/3 cup
- Wheat flour 2 cups
- Dry yeast 1 tsp.
- Salt 1 tsp.
- 1 tbsp. olive oil

Directions:

1. Pour the yeast with warm water. Stir the mixture properly so that there are no lumps.
2. Pour 2 cups flour and salt into a large bowl. Add yeast and knead the dough.
3. Put the dough out of the bowl on a dry, floured surface, and continue to knead, adding flour if

necessary, until the dough is soft and elastic (about 10 minutes).

4.   Lightly grease a large bowl with olive oil. Put the dough in a bowl, turning it so that the entire surface is smeared with oil.

5.   Cover with a film and place in a warm, without drafts, place for 1.5 hours (until the dough increases about 2 times).

6.   Flatten the dough with your fists. Divide into 2 parts and roll into balls.

Nutrition:

Calories: 392;

Protein: 8.3g;

Carbs: 44g;

Fat: 6.3g

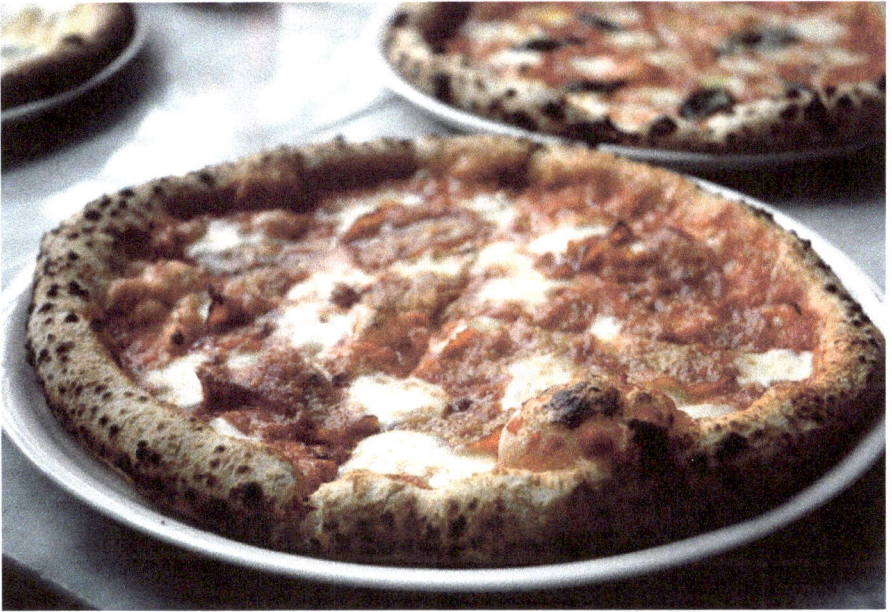

Crispy Pizza Dough

Preparation Time: 10 minutes

Cooking Time: 25 minutes

Servings: 5

Ingredients:

- Wheat flour 2 cups
- 2 tbsp. olive oil
- ½ cup milk
- Chicken egg 2 pieces
- Salt pinch

Directions:

1. Heat milk, add eggs and butter, stir.
2. Constantly mixing, pour the milk mixture into the flour, add salt
3. Knead the dough for about 10 minutes to make it elastic.

Nutrition:

Calories: 253;

Protein: 9.3g;

Carbs: 34g;

Fat: 6.3g

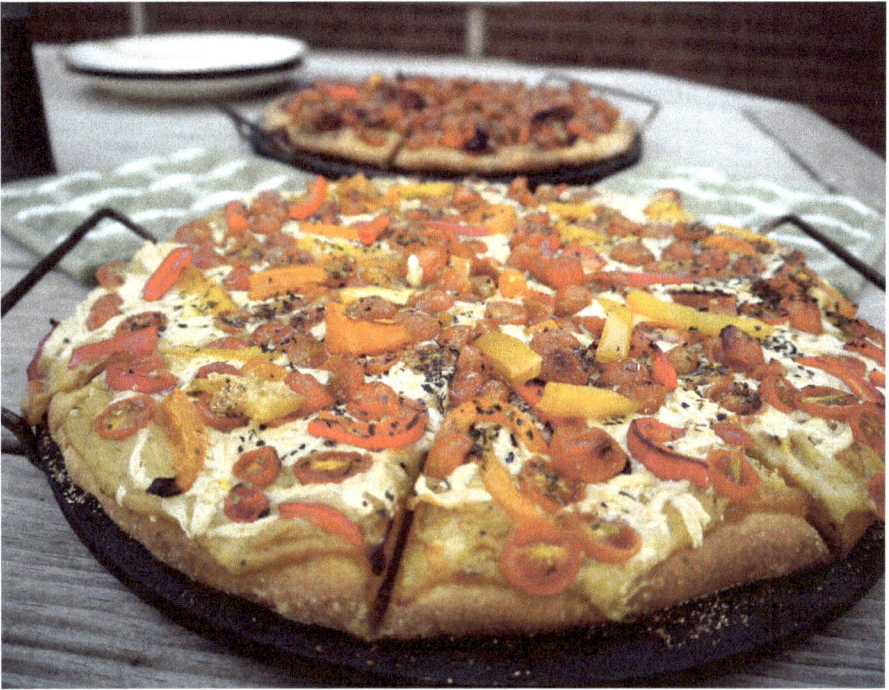

Thin Crispy Pizza Dough

Preparation Time: 10 minutes

Cooking Time: 20 minutes

Servings:

Ingredients:

- Wheat flour 9 oz.
- Cane sugar 0.3 tsp.
- Dry yeast 4 g
- 0.4 tsp. salt
- Water 125 ml

Directions:

1. Prepare the dough. To do this, mix yeast, sugar and 2 tbsp. of warm water in a bowl. Then add 2 tbsp. of flour, mix well again, cover with a towel and put in a warm place for 30 minutes. Watch the dough, it happens that it is ready in 10 minutes!

2. Pour flour into a bowl, make a depression in the middle. Put the dough in the recess, salt, add about 125 ml of warm water. Knead for about 10-15 minutes until the dough is soft, smooth and elastic. It should not stick to your hands, so you may need to add a little flour or water.

3. Cover the dough with a towel and put in a warm place for 1 hour. It should increase in volume by about half.

4. Making a crunch! Heat the oven to 350°F, grease the pizza dish with olive oil, roll it out with a diameter of about 28 cm, put it in the mold, form the sides (or not), grease with tomato sauce and put in the oven for about 5 minutes.

5. Then remove, distribute the rest of the filling and bake for another 20 minutes. Due to the fact that the dough is slightly baked at the beginning, it will become crispy, but at the same time it will not burn!

Nutrition:

Calories: 233;

Protein: 10.3g;

Carbs: 34g;

Fat: 5.3g

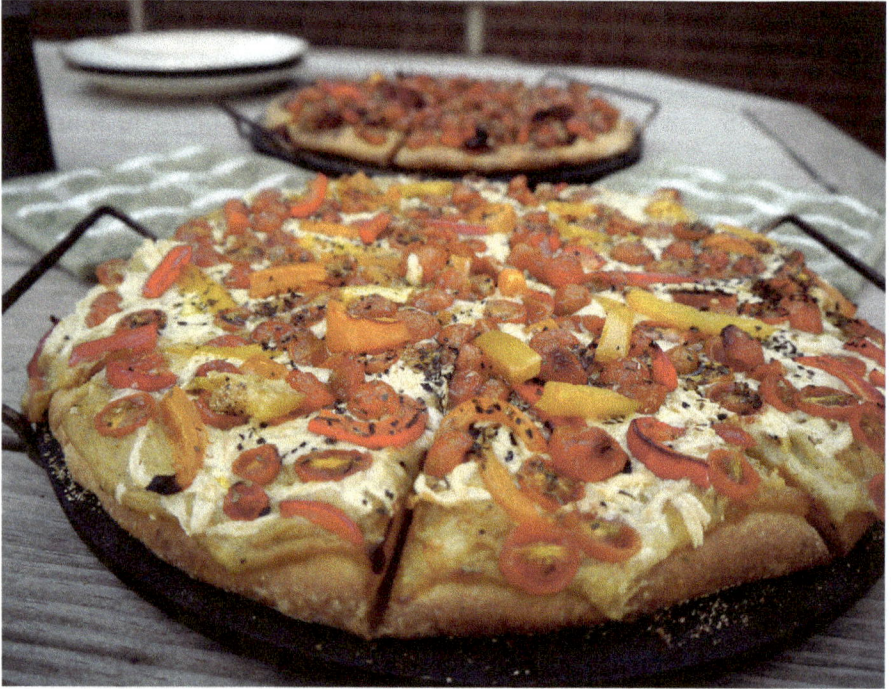

Yeast Pizza Dough

Preparation Time: 10 minutes

Cooking Time: 15 minutes

Servings: 5

Ingredients:

- Wheat flour 2 cups
- Vegetable oil 1 tbsp.
- Fresh yeast 3/4 oz.
- Sugar 1 tsp.
- Salt 1 tsp.

Directions:

1. In one glass of warm water, dilute 3/4 oz. of yeast (or 1/3 sachet of dry yeast). Leave to stand for 10 minutes.
2. Add 1 tbsp. of vegetable oil, pour all this into 2 cups flour, add salt and sugar.
3. Knead the dough well.

Nutrition:

Calories: 353;

Protein: 10.3g;

Carbs: 34g;

Fat: 5.3g

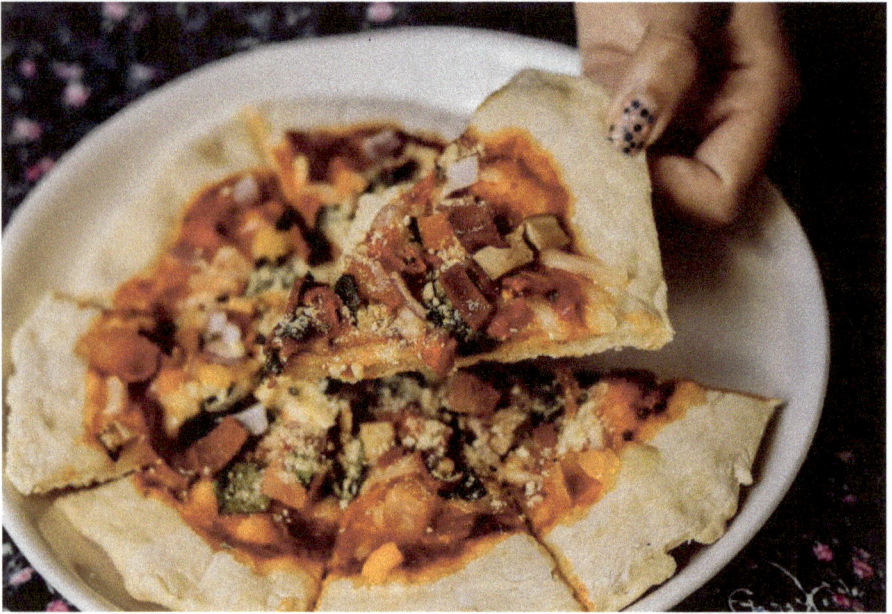

Fresh Sour Cream Pizza Dough

Preparation Time: 10 minutes

Cooking Time: 15 minutes

Servings: 5

Ingredients:

- Wheat flour 7 oz.
- Sour cream 7 oz.

Directions:

1. Knead the dough from flour and sour cream, divide into 3 equal parts, roll each part into a thin circle.
2. Put on a baking sheet, put the filling.

Nutrition:

Calories: 333;

Protein: 10.3g;

Carbs: 21.4g;

Fat: 12.3g

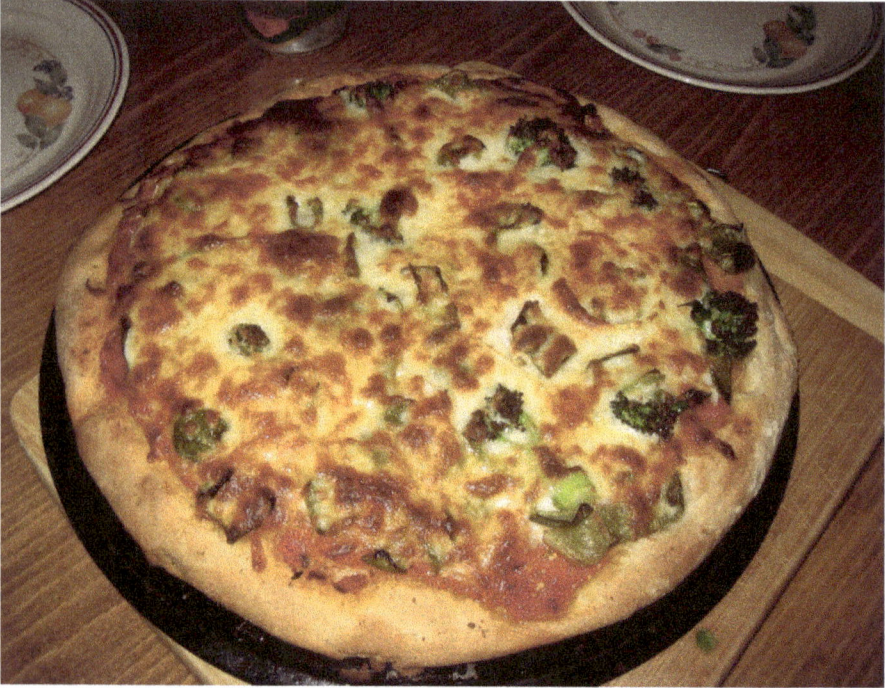

Fast, Yeast-Free Pizza Dough

Preparation Time: 10 minutes

Cooking Time: 25 minutes

Servings: 3

Ingredients:

- Wheat flour 12 oz.
- Kefir 250 ml
- Chicken egg 2 pieces
- Olive oil 40 ml
- ¼ tsp. salt
- ¼ tsp. soda

Directions:

1. Beat eggs with salt in a small bowl.
2. Pour kefir into a large bowl.
3. Add to the kefir soda quenched with vinegar.
4. Pour beaten eggs to kefir, mix well the mixture.

5. Add the flour, I prefer to add it in parts to feel the consistency of the dough. In principle, you can use a blender to prepare the dough, but I prefer to knead this particular dough with my hands.
6. Add olive oil to the dough.
7. Stir the dough. It should be consistency like thick sour cream - liquid, but at the same time it should turn out magnificent - as a result of the reaction of kefir and soda.
8. Lubricate the baking sheet with vegetable oil and pour the quick pizza dough on kefir and put the baking sheet in the oven about 400°F. When the dough is browned, you can spread the filling and bake until cooked.

Nutrition:

Calories: 468;

Protein: 20.3g;

Carbs: 41g;

Fat: 15.3g

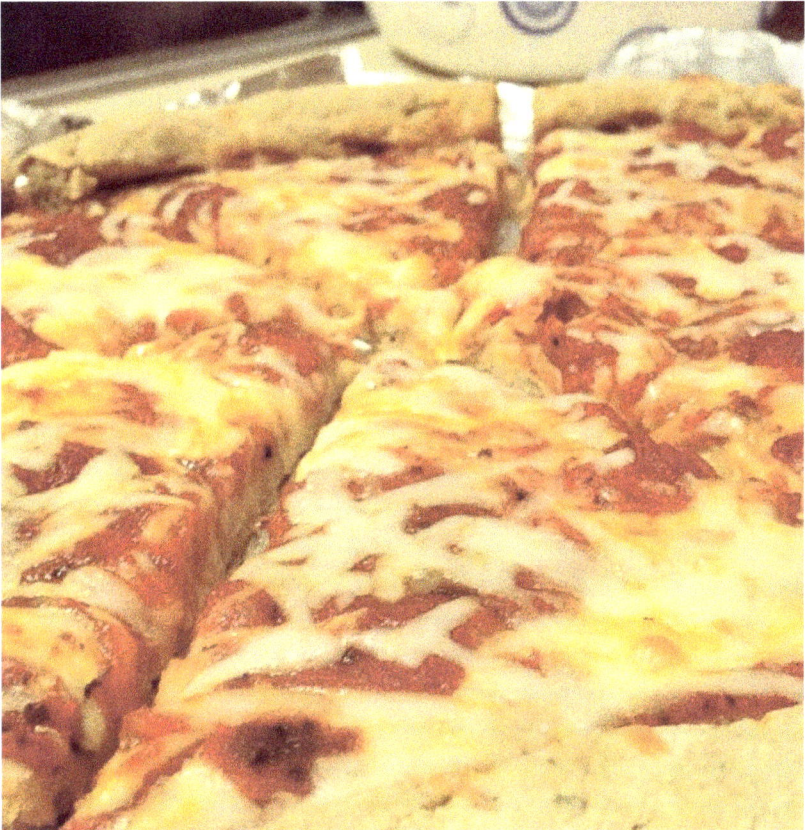

Thin Pizza Dough With Honey

Preparation Time: 10 minutes

Cooking Time: 15 minutes

Servings: 5

Ingredients:

- Wheat flour 3 cups
- Water 1 cup
- Dry yeast 12 g
- Honey 1.5 tsp.
- Salt 1 tsp.
- 1 tbsp. olive oil

Directions:

1. Heat the water to 120°F. Combine half a glass of warm water with yeast (12 g - 1 sachet) and honey.
2. Separately mix flour, salt, oil.

3. Add the honey-yeast mixture and the remaining water. Knead for at least 5 minutes (the dough should not stick to your hands).
4. Allow the dough to rise in a warm place for 30 minutes (cover with a damp towel so that the dough is not weathered).
5. Knead the dough again for 2 minutes, roll into a circle about 30 cm and put on a baking sheet, pre-oiled. The filling is your choice.

Nutrition:

Calories: 386;

Protein: 10.3g;

Carbs: 6.6g;

Fat: 4.3g

Pasta (Pizza Dough)

Preparation Time: 10 minutes

Cooking Time: 20 minutes

Servings: 4

Ingredients:

- Wheat flour 17 oz.
- Salt ¼ oz.
- Sugar ½ oz.
- Water 300 ml
- Olive oil 50 ml
- Dry yeast 7g

Directions:

1. Mix the dry ingredients: flour, salt and sugar.
2. In another bowl, mix water (room temperature), yeast and oil.
3. Combine everything and knead the dough.
4. Leave the dough for an hour, cover with a towel.
5. Distribute on a baking sheet, form the base of the pizza.
6. Lubricate with tomato paste, sprinkle with grated mozzarella and fill the pizza as desired (very tasty with mushrooms and prosciutto, or with tuna and olives), garnish with basil leaves.
7. Bake at 390°F for approximately 20–25 minutes.

Nutrition:

Calories: 562;

Protein: 10.3g;

Carbs: 3.4g;

Fat: 14.3g

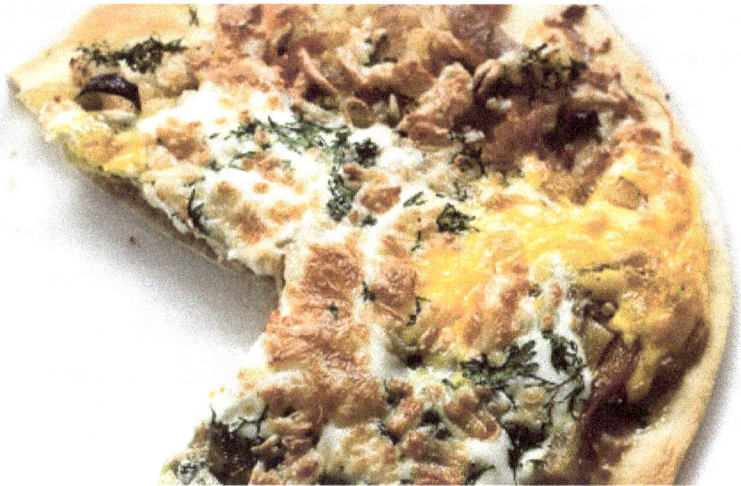

Pizza Dough Without Yeast In Milk

Preparation Time: 5 minutes

Cooking Time: 1 hour

Servings: 5

Ingredients:

- Wheat flour 2 cups
- Milk 125 ml
- Salt 1 tsp.
- Chicken egg 2 pieces
- Sunflower oil 2 tbsp.

Directions:

1. Making pizza dough without yeast in milk is quite simple. The recipe is designed to prepare a dough, which is enough for two, but only large, baking sheets.

2. Combine flour and salt in one bowl. And in the second butter, milk and eggs, mix well and combine the contents of two bowls in one large container.

3. Wait a few minutes for the whole liquid consistency to soak in the flour, and start mixing the dough. It will take about 15 minutes. Dough, in finished form, should be elastic, soft and smooth.

4. Then you need to take a kitchen towel, of course clean, and soak it in water. As a result, it should

be moist, but not wet. Excess fluid must be squeezed out. Wrap the dough in a towel, leave to lie down for 20 minutes.

5.   After waiting for the set time, remove the dough and, sprinkling flour on the countertop, roll out, but only very thinly.

6.   Place it on a baking sheet and lay out the filling prepared according to your taste preferences. As a result, the finished dough will have an effect that is easy, of course, of puff pastry and has a crispy taste.

Nutrition:

Calories: 453;

Protein: 10.3g;

Carbs: 30.4g;

Fat: 14.3g

Puff Pastry Pizza

Preparation Time: 10 minutes

Cooking Time: 30 minutes

Servings: 5

Ingredients:

- Puff pastry 17 oz.
- Sausages 7 oz.
- Hard cheese 5 oz.
- Tomatoes 4 pieces
- Dill 1 bunch
- Mayonnaise to taste
- Tomato paste to taste
- Champagne Vinegar 150 ml

Directions:

1. Thaw the dough, roll out, distribute on a baking sheet greased with vegetable oil, make small sides.
2. Sausages cut into rings. Cut the tomatoes into slices. Grate the cheese. Fry the champignons in a pan, add chopped herbs, mix.
3. Grease the dough with tomato paste, put sausages, then tomatoes, grease with mayonnaise, put mushrooms, sprinkle with cheese.
4. Put the pizza in the oven preheated to 360°F

Nutrition:

Calories: 253;

Protein: 10.3g;

Carbs: 3.4g;

Fat: 16.3g

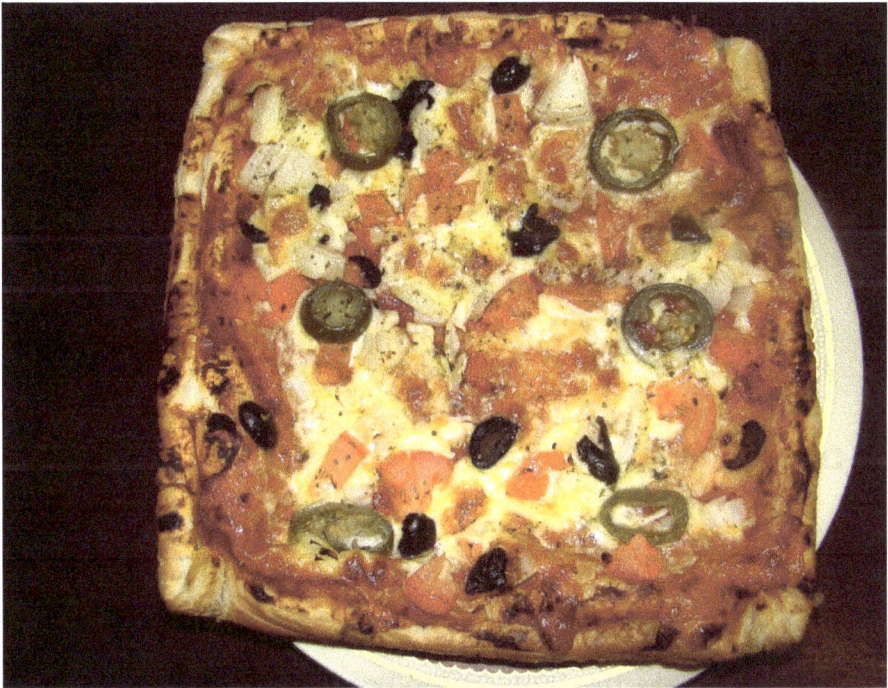

Ideal Pizza Dough (On A Large Baking Sheet)

Preparation Time: 10 minutes

Cooking Time: 1 hour

Servings: 5

Ingredients:

- Wheat flour 13 oz.
- Salt 1.5 tsp.
- Dry yeast 1,799 tsp.
- Sugar 1 tsp.
- Water 200 ml
- 1 tbsp. olive oil
- Dried Basil 1.5 tsp.

Directions:

1. We cultivate yeast in warm water. There you can add a spoonful of sugar, so the yeast will begin to work faster. Leave them for 10 minutes.
2. Sift the flour through a sieve (leave 2 oz. for the future) in a deep bowl. Add salt, basil, mix.
3. Pour water with yeast into the cavity in the flour and mix thoroughly with a fork.

4. Somewhere in the middle of the process, when the dough becomes less than one whole, add olive oil (you can also sunflower).

5. When the dough is ready (it becomes smooth and elastic), cover with a damp towel and put in heat (you can use the battery) for 30 minutes.

6. Now just lay it on a flour dusted surface and roll out the future pizza to a thickness of 2-3 mm.

7. The main rule of pizza is the maximum possible temperature, minimum time. Therefore, feel free to set the highest temperature that is available in your oven.

Nutrition:

Calories: 193;

Protein: 10.3g;

Carbs: 34g;

Fat: 9.3g

Vegetable Oil Pizza Dough

Preparation Time: 10 minutes

Cooking Time: 1 hour

Servings: 3

Ingredients:

- Wheat flour 1 cup
- Water 1 cup
- Salt to taste
- Vegetable oil 1 tbsp.
- Dry yeast 10 g

Directions:

1. We mix water and yeast, leave for 40 minutes so that they disperse. You can add a tbsp. of sugar.
2. Then pour in the oil, add the flour (here already at the request and degree of tightness of the dough - it should be quite tight, but not too much).
3. Knead well and put in a warm place to increase the volume by 2 times.

Nutrition:

Calories: 223;

Protein: 10.3g;

Carbs: 9.4g;

Fat: 5.3g

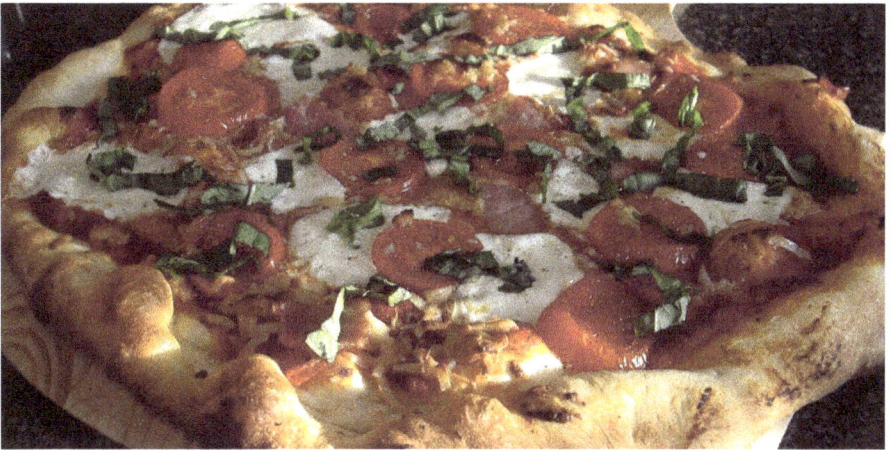

Pizza Dough On Yogurt

Preparation Time: 10 minutes

Cooking Time: 30 minutes

Servings: 5

Ingredients:

- Natural yogurt 9 oz.
- Vegetable oil 5 tbsp.
- ½ tsp. salt
- Wheat flour 2.5 cups
- Baking powder 1 tsp.

Directions:

1. Mix flour, baking powder and salt;
2. Add yogurt and butter, mix everything thoroughly;
3. Preheat the oven to 190 ° C;
4. Lubricate the pan with oil;
5. Roll the dough very thinly and transfer to a baking sheet;
6. Put the filling to taste;
7. Bake for 10-15 minutes.

Nutrition:

Calories: 336;

Protein: 10.3g;

Carbs: 24g;

Fat: 13.3g

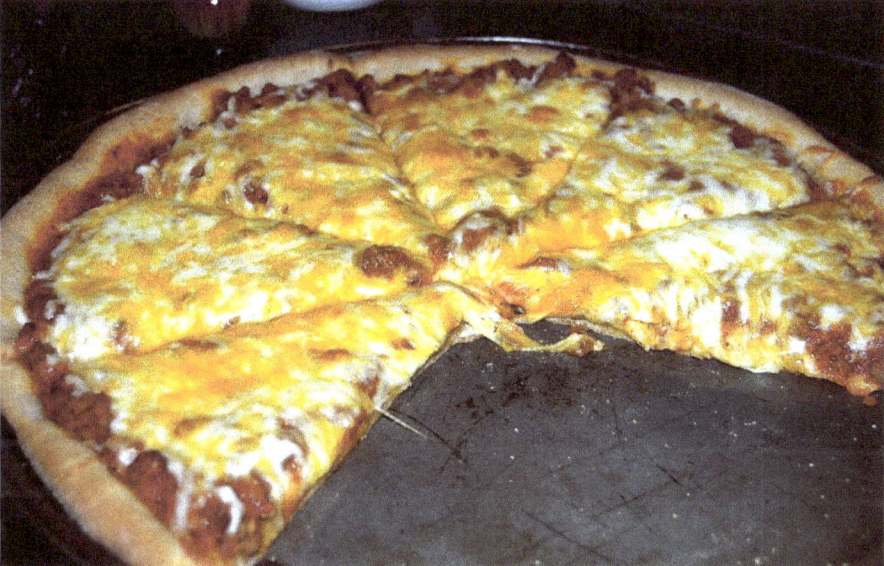

American Pizza Dough Recipe

Preparation Time: 10 minutes

Cooking Time: 15 minutes

Servings: 5

Ingredients:

- Wheat flour 6 oz.
- Chicken egg 1 piece
- Water 85 ml
- Dry yeast 2 g
- Salt 3 g
- Sugar 10 g
- Sunflower oil 5 ml

Directions:

1. Combine all dry ingredients.
2. Add water and egg. Mix well.
3. After the dough has become homogeneous, gradually add the butter.
4. Leave the dough for 5 minutes.

Nutrition:

Calories: 353;

Protein: 18.3g;

Carbs: 27g;

Fat: 13.3g

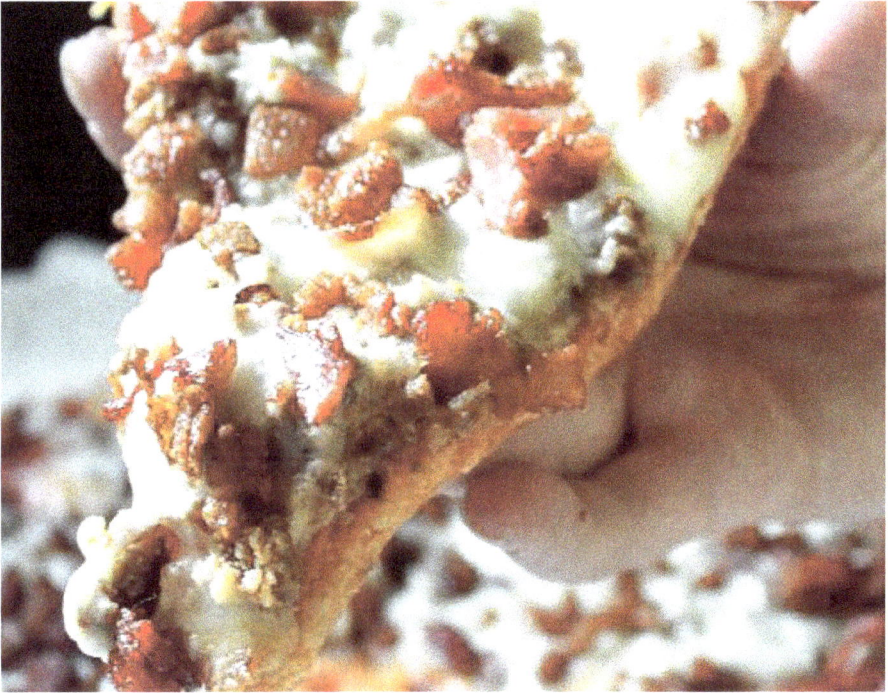

Eggplant Pizza

Preparation Time: 10 minutes

Cooking Time: 30 minutes

Servings: 6

Ingredients:

- Eggplants (1 large or 2 medium)
- Olive oil (.33 cup)
- Black pepper & salt (as desired)
- Marinara sauce - store-bought/homemade (1.25 cups)
- Shredded mozzarella cheese (1.5 cups)
- Cherry tomatoes (2 cups - halved)
- Torn basil leaves (.5 cup)

Directions:

1. Heat the oven to reach 400°F. Prepare a baking sheet with a layer of parchment baking paper.

2. Slice the end/ends off of the eggplant and them it into ¾-inch slices. Arrange the slices on the prepared sheet and brush both sides with olive oil. Dust with pepper and salt to your liking.

3. Roast the eggplant until tender (10 to 12 min.).

4. Transfer the tray from the oven and add two tbsp. of sauce on top of each section. Top it off with the mozzarella and three to five tomato pieces on top.

5. Bake it until the cheese is melted. The tomatoes should begin to blister in about five to seven more minutes.

6. Take the tray from the oven. Serve hot and garnish with a dusting of basil.

Nutrition:

 Protein: 8 g

Fat: 20 g

Carbs: 25 g

Calories: 257

Mediterranean Whole Wheat Pizza

Preparation Time: 5 minutes

Cooking Time: 25 minutes

Servings: 4

Ingredients:

- Whole-wheat pizza crust (1)
- Basil pesto (4 oz. jar)
- Artichoke hearts (.5 cup)
- Kalamata olives (2 tbsp.)
- Pepperoncini (2 tbsp. drained)
- Feta cheese (.25 cup)

Directions:

1. Program the oven to 450°F.
2. Drain and pull the artichokes to pieces. Slice/chop the pepperoncini and olives.
3. Arrange the pizza crust onto a floured work surface and cover it using pesto. Arrange the artichoke, pepperoncini slices, and olives over the pizza. Lastly, crumble and add the feta.
4. Bake in the hot oven until the cheese has melted, and it has a crispy crust or 10-12 minutes.

Nutrition:

Calories: 277

Protein: 9.7 g

Carbs: 24 g

Fat: 18.6 g

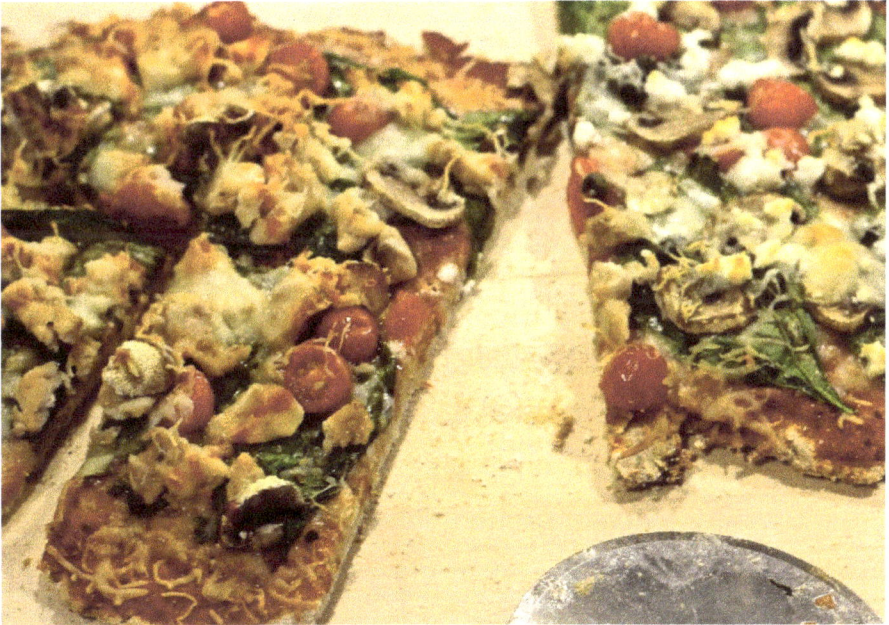

Chicken Pizza

Preparation Time: 1 minute

Cooking Time: 10 minutes

Servings: 4

Ingredients:

- 2 flatbreads
- 1 tbsp. Greek vinaigrette
- ½ cup feta cheese, crumbled
- ¼ cup Parmesan cheese, grated
- ½ cup water-packed artichoke hearts, rinsed, drained and chopped
- ½ cup olives, pitted and sliced
- ½ cup cooked chicken breast strips, chopped
- 1/8 tsp. dried basil
- 1/8 tsp. dried oregano
- Pinch of ground black pepper
- 1 cup part-skim mozzarella cheese, shredded

Directions:

1. Preheat the oven to 400°F.

2. Arrange the flatbreads onto a large ungreased baking sheet and coat each with vinaigrette.
3. Top with feta, followed by the Parmesan, veggies and chicken.
4. Sprinkle with dried herbs and black pepper.
5. Top with mozzarella cheese evenly.
6. Bake for about 8-10 minutes or until cheese is melted.
7. Remove from the oven and set aside for about 1-2 minutes before slicing.
8. Cut each flat bread into 2 pieces and serve.

Nutrition:

Calories 393

Fat 22 g

Carbs 20.6 g

Protein 28.9 g

Spinach & Feta Pita Bake

Preparation Time: 10 minutes

Cooking Time: 22 minutes

Servings: 6

Ingredients:

- Sun-dried tomato pesto (6 oz. tub)
- Roma - plum tomatoes (2 chopped)
- Whole-wheat pita bread (Six 6-inch)
- Spinach (1 bunch)
- Mushrooms (4 sliced)
- Grated Parmesan cheese (2 tbsp.)
- Crumbled feta cheese (.5 cup)
- Olive oil (3 tbsp.)
- Black pepper (as desired)

Directions:

1. Set the oven at 350°F.
2. Spread the pesto onto one side of each pita bread and arrange them onto a baking tray (pesto-side up).
3. Rinse and chop the spinach. Top the pitas with spinach, mushrooms, tomatoes, feta cheese, pepper, Parmesan cheese, pepper, and a drizzle of oil.

4. Bake in the hot oven until the pita bread is crispy
    (12 min.). Slice the pitas into quarters.

Nutrition:

Calories: 350

Protein: 11.6 g

Carbs: 24 g

Fat: 17.1g g

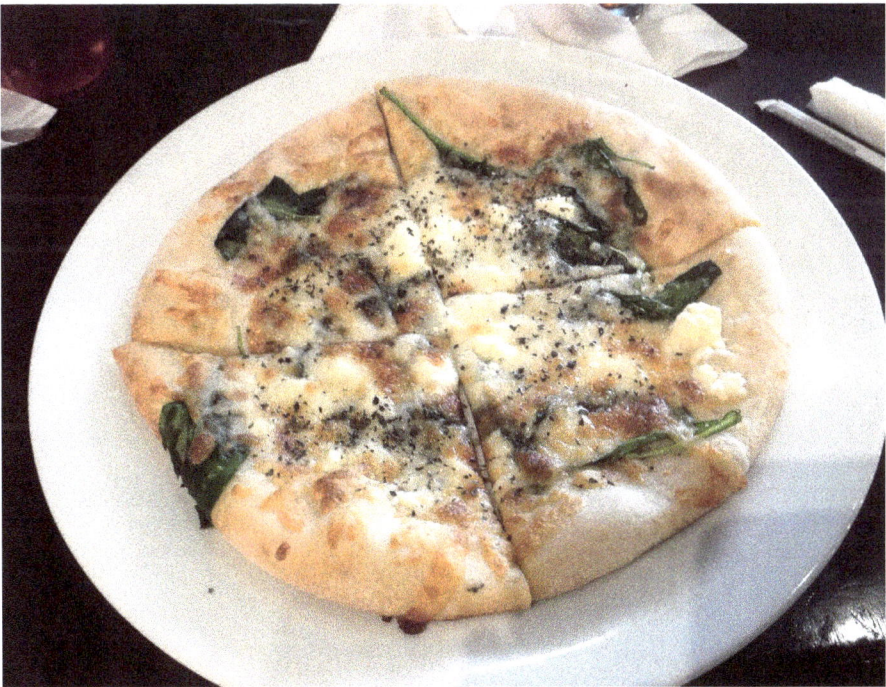

Beef Pizza

Preparation Time: 25 minutes

Cooking Time: 50 minutes

Servings: 10

Ingredients:

For Crust:

- 3 cups all-purpose flour
- 1 tbsp. sugar
- 2¼ tsp. active dry yeast
- 1 tsp. salt
- 2 tbsp. olive oil
- 1 cup warm water

For Topping:

- 1-lb. ground beef
- 1 medium onion, chopped
- 2 tbsp. tomato paste
- 1 tbsp. ground cumin
- Salt and ground black pepper, as required
- ¼ cup water
- 1 cup fresh spinach, chopped
- 8 oz. artichoke hearts, quartered

- 4 oz. fresh mushrooms, sliced
- 2 tomatoes, chopped
- 4 oz. feta cheese, crumbled

Directions:

For crust:

1. In the bowl of a stand mixer, fitted with the dough hook, add the flour, sugar, yeast and salt.
2. Add 2 tbsp. of the oil and warm water and knead until a smooth and elastic dough is formed.
3. Make a ball of the dough and set aside for about 15 minutes.
4. Place the dough onto a lightly floured surface and roll into a circle.
5. Place the dough into a lightly, greased round pizza pan and gently, press to fit.
6. Set aside for about 10-15 minutes.
7. Coat the crust with some oil.
8. Preheat the oven to 400°F.

For topping:

9. Heat a nonstick skillet over medium-high heat and cook the beef for about 4-5 minutes.
10. Add the onion and cook for about 5 minutes, stirring frequently.

11. Add the tomato paste, cumin, salt, black pepper and water and stir to combine.
12. Reduce the heat to medium and cook for about 5-10 minutes.
13. Remove from the heat and set aside.
14. Place the beef mixture over the pizza crust and top with the spinach, followed by the artichokes, mushrooms, tomatoes, and Feta cheese.
15. Bake for about 25-30 minutes or until the cheese is melted.
16. Remove from the oven and set aside for about 3-5 minutes before slicing.
17. Cut into desired sized slices and serve.

Nutrition:

Calories 309

Fat 8.7 g

Carbs 36.4 g

Protein 21.4 g

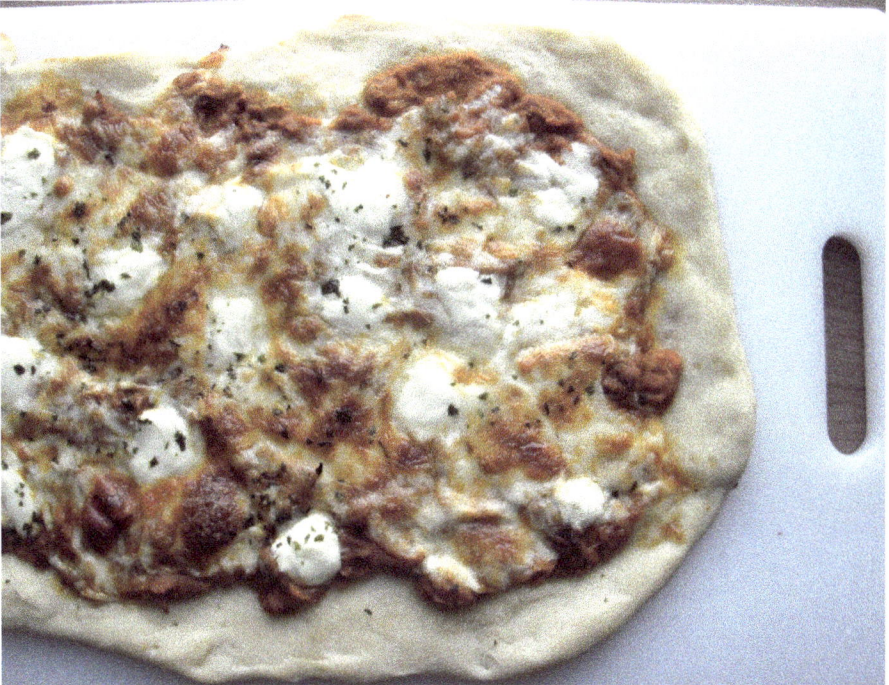

Shrimp Pizza

Preparation Time: 15 minutes

Cooking Time: 10 minutes

Servings: 1

Ingredients:

- 2 tbsp. spaghetti sauce
- 1 tbsp. pesto sauce
- 1 (6-inch) pita bread
- 2 tbsp. mozzarella cheese, shredded
- 5 cherry tomatoes, halved
- 1/8 cup bay shrimp
- Pinch of garlic powder
- Pinch of dried basil

Directions:

1. Preheat the oven to 325°F. Lightly, grease a baking sheet.
2. In a bowl, mix together the spaghetti sauce and pesto.

3. Spread the pesto mixture over the pita bread in a thin layer.

4. Top the pita bread with the cheese, followed by the tomatoes and shrimp.

5. Sprinkle with the garlic powder and basil.

6. Arrange the pita bread onto the prepared baking sheet and bake for about 7-10 minutes.

7. Remove from the oven and set aside for about 3-5 minutes before slicing.

8. Cut into desired sized slices and serve.

Nutrition:

Calories 482

Fat 18.9 g

Carbs 44.5 g

Protein 33.4 g

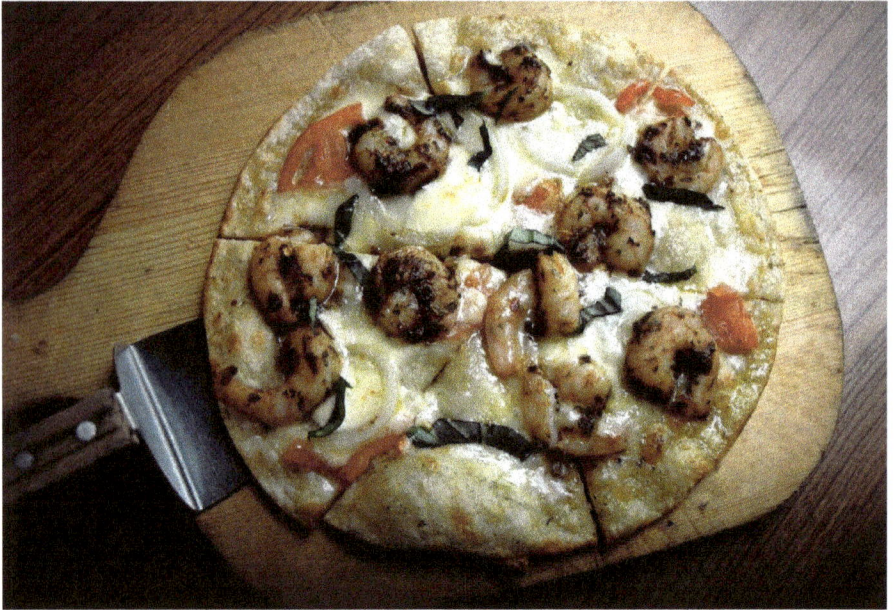

Veggie Pizza

Preparation Time: 20 minutes

Cooking Time: 12 minutes

Servings: 6

Ingredients:

- 1 (12-inch) prepared pizza crust
- ¼ tsp. Italian seasoning
- ¼ tsp. red pepper flakes, crushed
- 1 cup goat cheese, crumbled
- 1 (14-oz.) can quartered artichoke hearts
- 3 plum tomatoes, sliced into ¼-inch thick size
- 6 kalamata olives, pitted and sliced
- ¼ cup fresh basil, chopped

Directions:

1. Preheat the oven to 450°F. Grease a baking sheet.
2. Sprinkle the pizza crust with Italian seasoning and red pepper flakes evenly.
3. Place the goat cheese over crust evenly, leaving about ½-inch of the sides.
4. With the back of a spoon, gently press the cheese downwards.

5. Place the artichoke, tomato and olives on top of the cheese.
6. Arrange the pizza crust onto the prepared baking sheet.
7. Bake for about 10-12 minutes or till cheese becomes bubbly.
8. Remove from oven and sprinkle with the basil.
9. Cut into equal sized wedges and serve.

Nutrition:

Calories 381

Fat 16.1 g

Carbs 42.4 g

Protein 19.4 g

Watermelon Feta & Balsamic Pizza

Preparation Time: 5 minutes

Cooking Time: 15 minutes

Servings: 4

Ingredients:

- Watermelon (1-inch thick from the center)
- Crumbled feta cheese (1 oz.)
- Sliced Kalamata olives (5-6)
- Mint leaves (1 tsp.)
- Balsamic glaze (.5 tbsp.)

Directions:

1. Slice the widest section of the watermelon in half. Then, slice each half into four wedges.
2. Serve on a round pie dish like a pizza round and cover with the olives, cheese, mint leaves, and glaze.

Nutrition:

Calories: 90

Protein: 2 g

Fat: 3 g

Carbs 5 g

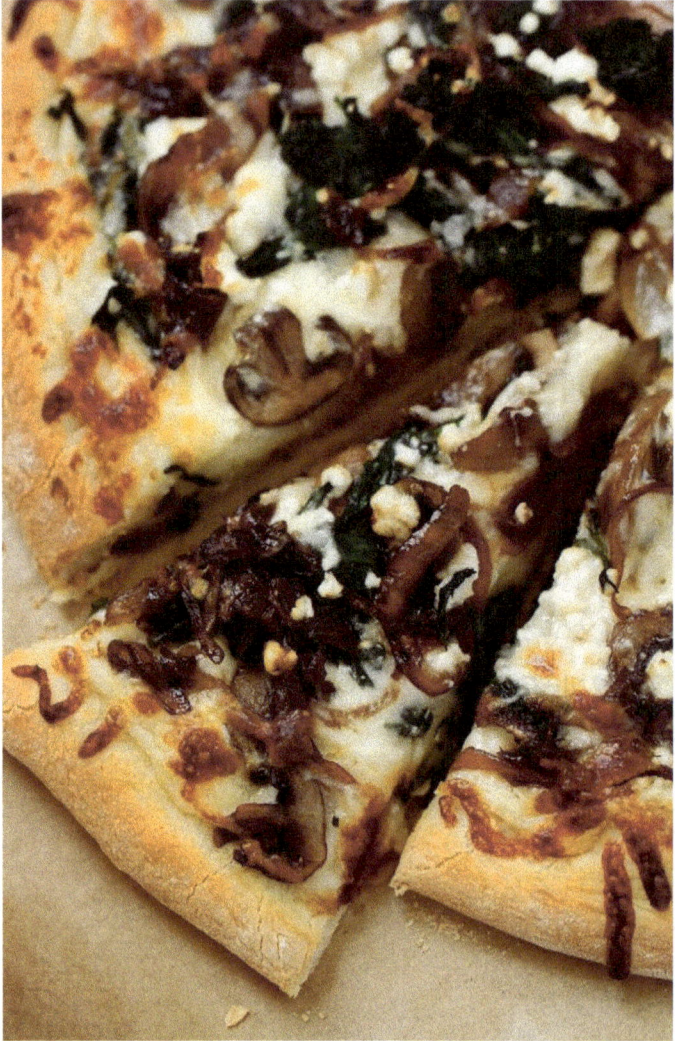

Fruit Pizza

Preparation Time: 15 minutes

Cooking Time: 0 minutes

Servings: 4

Ingredients:

- 4 watermelon slices
- 1 oz blueberries
- 2 oz goat cheese, crumbled
- 1 tsp. fresh parsley, chopped

Directions:

1. Put the watermelon slices in the plate in one layer.
2. Then sprinkle them with blueberries, goat cheese, and fresh parsley.

Nutrition: 69 Calories, 4.4g Protein, 1.4g Carbs, 5.1g Fat

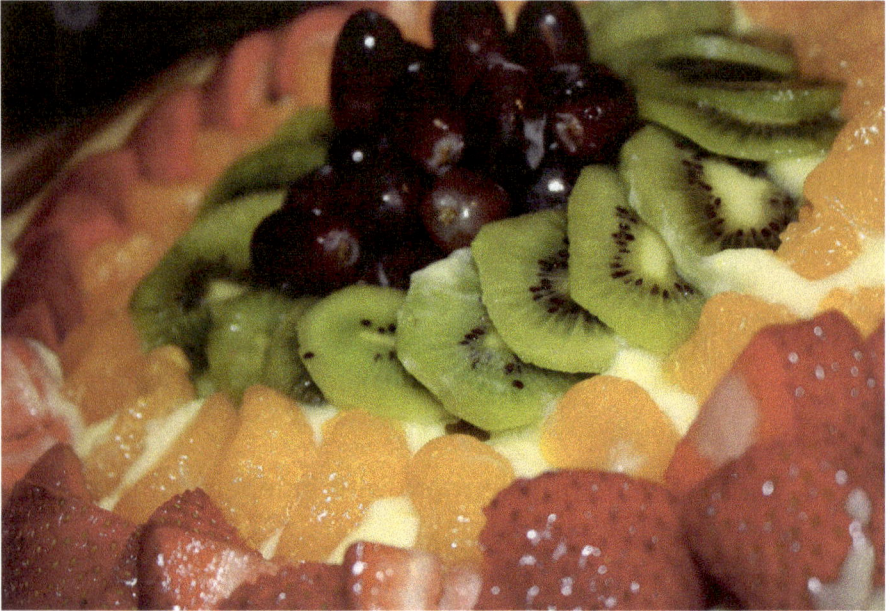

Sprouts Pizza

Preparation Time: 25 minutes

Cooking Time: 15 minutes

Servings: 6

Ingredients:

- 4 oz wheat flour, whole grain
- 2 tbsp. olive oil
- ¼ tsp. baking powder
- 5 oz chicken fillet, boiled
- 2 oz Mozzarella cheese, shredded
- 1 tomato, chopped
- 2 oz bean sprouts

Directions:

1. Make the pizza crust: mix wheat flour, olive oil, baking powder, and knead the dough.
2. Roll it up in the shape of pizza crust and transfer in the pizza mold.
3. Then sprinkle it with chopped tomato, shredded chicken, and Mozzarella.
4. Bake the pizza at 365F for 15 minutes.
5. Sprinkle the cooked pizza with bean sprouts and cut into servings.

Nutrition: 184 Calories,11.9g Protein, 15.6g Carbs, 8.2g Fat

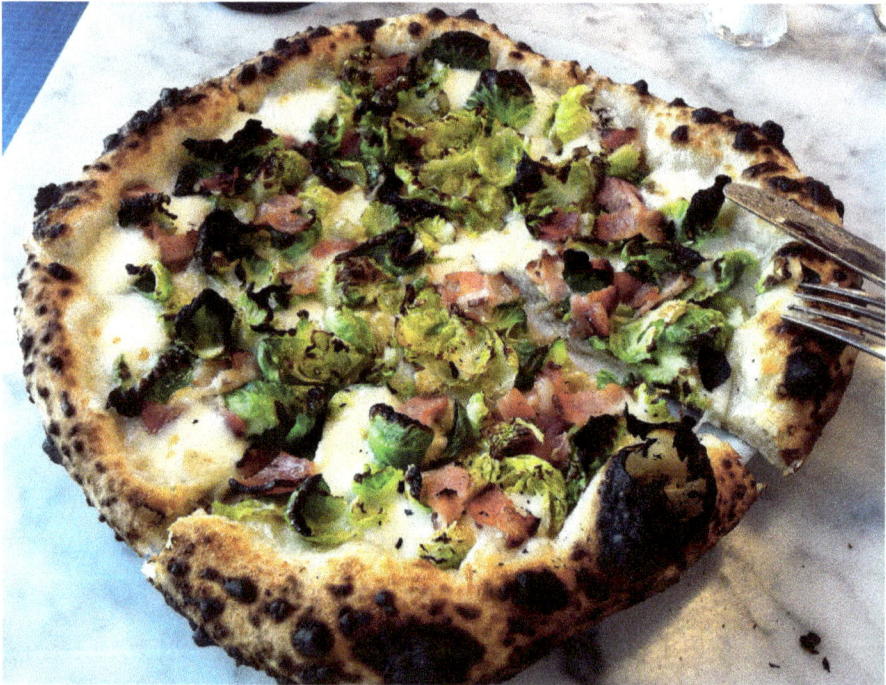

www.ingramcontent.com/pod-product-compliance
Lightning Source LLC
Chambersburg PA
CBHW050752030426

42336CB00012B/1777